D1258065

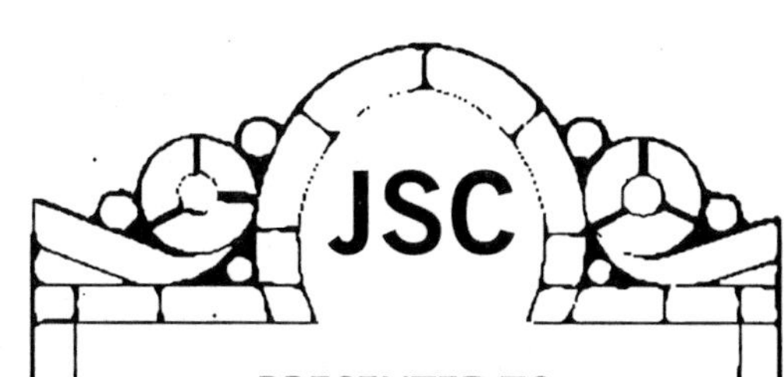
JSC

Childhood Mental Health Disorders

Childhood Mental Health Disorders

Evidence Base and Contextual Factors for Psychosocial, Psychopharmacological, and Combined Interventions

Ronald T. Brown

David O. Antonuccio

George J. DuPaul

Mary A. Fristad

Cheryl A. King

Laurel K. Leslie

Gabriele S. McCormick

William E. Pelham Jr.

John C. Piacentini

Benedetto Vitiello

American Psychological Association
Washington, DC

Published by
American Psychological Association
750 First Street, NE
Washington, DC 20002
www.apa.org

To order
APA Order Department
P.O. Box 92984
Washington, DC 20090-2984
Tel: (800) 374-2721; Direct: (202) 336-5510
Fax: (202) 336-5502; TDD/TTY: (202) 336-6123
Online: www.apa.org/books/
E-mail: order@apa.org

In the U.K., Europe, Africa, and the Middle East, copies may be ordered from
American Psychological Association
3 Henrietta Street
Covent Garden, London
WC2E 8LU England

Typeset in Goudy by Stephen McDougal, Mechanicsville, MD

Printer: Edwards Brothers, Inc., Ann Arbor, MI
Cover Designer: Go! Creative, Kensington, MD
Technical/Production Editor: Devon Bourexis

The opinions and statements published are the responsibility of the authors, and such opinions and statements do not necessarily represent the policies of the American Psychological Association.

Library of Congress Cataloging-in-Publication Data

Childhood mental health disorders : evidence base and contextual factors for psychosocial, psychopharmacological, and combined interventions / Ronald T. Brown [et al.].
p. ; cm.
Includes bibliographical references.
ISBN-13: 978-1-4338-0170-9
ISBN-10: 1-4338-0170-1
1. Child psychopathology. 2. Child psychopathology—Treatment. 3. Child psychopathology—Chemotherapy. I. Brown, Ronald T.
[DNLM: 1. Child. 2. Mental Disorders—therapy. 3. Adolescent. 4. Psychotherapy—methods. 5. Psychotropic Drugs—therapeutic use. 6. Review Literature. WS 350 C53788 2008]

RJ499.C4875 2008
618.92'89—dc22 2007012594

British Library Cataloguing-in-Publication Data
A CIP record is available from the British Library.

Printed in the United States of America
First Edition

CONTENTS

FOREWORD

THOMAS OLLENDICK

The marriage of molecular neuroscience and cognitive psychology is driving a revolution in how we understand the diagnosis, assessment, and treatment of childhood and adolescent mental disorders. It is now evident that these disorders are highly complex, multiply determined, and embedded in rich social, cultural, familial, and developmental contexts. Moreover, it is becoming increasingly clear that a complete or full conceptualization of these disorders can be captured best by what has become known as the *developmental psychopathology perspective*—a perspective in which it is acknowledged that multiple pathways can lead to any one disorder (i.e., equifinality) and that any one pathway or set of pathways can result in multiple and diverse outcomes (i.e., multifinality). It is also increasingly clear that treatments for these disorders work in complex, interactive ways; for example, it is now generally accepted that psychotropic medications work, at least in part, by biasing specific central nervous system information-processing systems and that, similarly, psychosocial treatments work not only by the cognitive and behavioral balance they engender but also by their strong effects on the somatic substrate of the treated child.[1] Put simply, drugs and psychotherapy work at least in part because they act on the brain.[2] Hence, when selecting a treatment strategy that is appropriate to the needs of children or adolescents

[1]March, J. S., & Ollendick, T. H. (2004). Integrated psychosocial and pharmacological treatment. In T. H. Ollendick & J. S. March (Eds.), *Phobic and anxiety disorders in children and adolescents: A clinician's guide to effective psychosocial and pharmacological interventions* (pp. 141–172). New York: Oxford University Press.

[2]Hyman, S. E. (2000). The millennium of mind, brain, and behavior. *Archives of General Psychiatry*, 57, 88–89.

with a variety of disorders, the treating clinician must consider both medication and psychosocial treatment strategies, either alone or in combination with one another.

In a perfectly evidence-based world, selecting an appropriate treatment from among the many available possibilities would be reasonably straightforward. However, in the complex world of clinical practice, choices are rarely so clear-cut. Even when a comprehensive assessment produces an unambiguous diagnosis and clearly defined target symptoms, expected outcomes vary by factors specific to the treatment modality chosen; the clinician; the setting in which the treatment occurs; and, not least of all, the child and her or his social–developmental–familial context. Thus, the delivery of evidence-based practices in real-world settings is complex, and paint-by-number or cookie-cutter approaches will not suffice.

It is against this complex reality that the present volume produced by the American Psychological Association's (APA's) Working Group on Psychotropic Medications for Children and Adolescents has emerged. The working group, composed of eminent clinical child and adolescent psychologists and psychiatrists, has produced a volume that is comprehensive, scholarly, up-to-date, and sensitive to and responsive toward real-world clinical practice. Although the available evidence for which interventions to use in treating the various psychiatric disorders of childhood and adolescence is uneven and somewhat sketchy at times, the working group—consisting of members with considerable clinical acumen and experience—provides practitioners a set of working guidelines on what treatments to use for what problems and, assuming sufficient evidence exists, when to use combined pharmacological and psychosocial treatments. The state of the science is not exact, however, and the specific treatments chosen also need to be informed by child and family values. This all seems appropriate inasmuch as most accepted definitions of evidence-based practice include the integration of the best available evidence, the clinical experience and expertise of the treating clinician, and the values or preferences of the treated family.

Although considerable evidence and clinical experience support the therapeutic benefits of psychosocial and pharmacological interventions for the treatment of children and adolescents with mental disorders, it is also evident that much remains to be learned before we can be content with the current state of affairs. For example, we really do not know how well these evidence-based treatments work with children and adolescents who vary in age, gender, culture, race, and socioeconomic status. These moderators of treatment, along with others such as parental rearing practices and parental psychopathology, are only beginning to be specified, and our knowledge is sparse at this time. Addressing these issues will give us a clearer picture about the conditions under which these treatments work. Moreover, we really do not know much about the mechanisms of how or why these treatments work—we simply know that they tend to work. Understanding mechanisms of action might help us streamline the approaches and perhaps make them even more effective and efficient. In addition, we do not yet fully know how they work in various clinical settings or how to sequence the treatments when both psychosocial and pharmacological treatments appear warranted. Finally, the evidence is sparse on the long-term effectiveness of the various approaches and how well they address functional in addition to symptomatic outcomes. Obviously, much remains to be learned.

Still, it is evident from this volume that much has been accomplished, and we know a lot already. The working group nicely brings this information together for us in this volume. APA is to be commended for sponsoring this project and ushering it through to its completion. Along with its 2005 *Policy Statement on Evidence-Based Practice in Psychology*,[3] APA has taken its rightful stand on such issues and joined the forces of other organizations in identifying, promulgating, and disseminating such practices. The children and adolescents we serve surely deserve the best of what we have to offer them.

---

[3]American Psychological Association. (2005). *Policy statement on evidence-based practice in psychology*. Retrieved May 30, 2005, from http://www2.apa.org/practice/ebpstatement.pdf

PREFACE

Determining the appropriate treatments for children and adolescents has never been more challenging for mental health care providers and caregivers. The unstable nature of developments surrounding pharmaceuticals, resulting in advisories and black-box warnings, complicates any decision-making process. Most recently, issues of the safety of psychotropics have assumed prominence in the media as well as in scholarly literature. As a result, practitioners often find themselves confused with regard to the relative efficacy of various therapies. Further, they must balance the issue of efficacy with safety.

Against this dynamic backdrop, the American Psychological Association commissioned the Working Group on Psychotropic Medications for Children and Adolescents. The subgroup consisted of nine individuals, seven of whom were psychologists and two of whom were physicians (i.e., a pediatrician and a child and adolescent psychiatrist). Each individual brought a great deal of expertise to the group in various areas of psychopathology (e.g., attention-deficity/hyperactivity disorders, autism spectrum disorder, major depressive disorder, bipolar disorder), psychopharmacology (e.g., stimulants, antidepressants, neuroleptics), psychosocial treatments (e.g., behavior management, cognitive behavior therapy), health services research, and ethical issues pertaining to psychopharmacology. Members were selected by the committee because of their nationally recognized reputations as experts in their respective fields. Our working group was charged with reviewing the literature and preparing a comprehensive report on the current effective use, sequencing, and integration of psychotropic medications and psychosocial interventions for children and adolescents. A comparative examination of the risk–benefit ratio of psychosocial and pharmacological treatments and the extent of child and adolescent psychopharmacology, including the appropriateness of medication use, are part of the information presented.

The quick and constant changes in research in this field were challenging in preparing such a text. We made every attempt to include the most recent data, yet we fully acknowledge and remind the reader of the rapidly increasing and changing literature on psychopharmacological and psychosocial treatments for children and adolescents. This book represents a snapshot in time. A compendium such as this provides a starting point for understanding the science and practice of pediatric psychopharmacology in the context of psychosocial approaches to treatment. It also allows us to move toward addressing questions critical to the psychological well-being of children, adolescents, and their families. Our book is not the definitive word on these issues, but it can certainly be a basic yet comprehensive framework to guide mental health care providers and families as they attempt to improve the quality of life for children and adolescents. Although the World Wide Web has frequently become a major source of information for many families and consumers, this book offers a unique compendium of both psychopharmacological and psychosocial treatments and provides the strength of evidence for each of the treatments reviewed.

Even though we caution against using this volume as the definitive word, it is the opinion of the working group that the decision about which treatment to use first be in general guided by the balance between anticipated benefits and possible harms of treatment choices (including absence of treatment) that would be the most favorable to the child. This means practitioners should consider the safest treatments with demonstrated efficacy before considering other treatments with less favorable profiles. For most of the disorders reviewed herein, there are psychosocial treatments that are solidly grounded in empirical support as stand-alone treatments. Moreover, the preponderance of available evidence indicates that psychosocial treatments are safer than psychoactive medications. Thus, it is our recommendation that in most cases psychosocial interventions be considered first.

This book could not have been accomplished without the unwavering support and efforts of Mary Campbell. Her steadfast guidance and fruitful labor with the working group are interwoven throughout this book and were instrumental in its quality.

Childhood Mental Health Disorders

1

INTRODUCTION

The prevalence of child and adolescent mental disorders has been increasingly recognized. Also receiving increasing attention is the substantial morbidity associated with these child and adolescent mental disorders. In particular, the *Report of the Surgeon General's Conference on Children's Mental Health: A National Action Agenda* (U.S. Public Health Service, 2000) renewed public attention and identified children's mental health as a national priority. Prevalence estimates for childhood mental disorders in the United States range from 17.6% to 22% (Costello, Mustillo, Erkanli, Keeler, & Angold, 2003), which includes up to 15% of children and adolescents with a mental disorder severe enough to impair functioning (Roberts, Atkinson, & Rosenblatt, 1998; Shaffer, Fisher, Dulcan, & Davies, 1996). Of these 15%, data indicate that only 1 in 5 children receive services provided by appropriately trained mental health professionals (Burns et al., 1995; Centers for Disease Control and Prevention, 2004; U.S. Department of Health and Human Services, 1999). The renewed interest and increased recognition of mental disorders in children and adolescents have been paralleled by increased psychotropic medication prescriptions for children (Zito et al., 2002). This increase has led to closer public and scientific scrutiny of the efficacy and safety of these medications.

Driven by this increased attention, the number of scientific studies of treatment efficacy with children has risen dramatically (Vitiello, 2006). Support for pediatric treatment research is demonstrated by an increase in program announcements and requests for applications from the National Institutes of Health. As a result of congressional legislation in the 1990s, an approximate threefold increase in the proportion of the National Institute of Mental Health funding levels for clinical trials paralleled an increase in pharmaceutical company-sponsored clinical trials (Vitiello, Heiligenstein, Riddle, Greenhill, & Fegert, 2004). There was also a concurrent increase in research investigating several modalities. Several recent federally sponsored clinical trials have addressed the efficacy of psychosocial, psychopharmacologic, and combined interventions for childhood disorders.

Prompted by growing public recognition, research efforts are increasingly focusing on issues of safety and efficacy in treatment of mental health disorders in youth. Since the first use of psychotropic medication in children in the 1930s, safety questions have been present (R. T. Brown & Sammons, 2002). For example, concerns were raised in the 1970s about the use of stimulants for attention-deficit/hyperactivity disorder (ADHD; S. G. O'Leary, 1980). The same attention was applied to selective serotonin reuptake inhibitors (SSRIs) when they emerged in the early 1990s (R. A. King et al., 1991). These issues have more recently reached public awareness, especially the use of psychotropic medications for the treatment of depression in children and adolescents. The 2003 decision by the United Kingdom to define the use of most antidepressants as contraindicated in children (Whittington, Kendall, & Pilling, 2005) was followed by scrutiny of safety data from clinical trials in the United States, and the U.S. Food and Drug Administration (FDA) mandated caution and warning about these medications.

Given this changing landscape, the working group on psychotropic medications for children and adolescents worked to provide an up-to-date and comprehensive review of the state of knowledge of the effective use, sequencing, and integration of psychotropic medications and psychosocial interventions. Psychosocial interventions in this book represent the range of treatments across populations (e.g., youths, families, teachers) and across areas of functioning. Psychosocial interventions are both the evidence-based alternatives and complementary interventions to medications. Medications cannot be appropriately evaluated without considering the alternatives. This book contains a comparative examination of the risk–benefit ratio of psychosocial, psychopharmacological, and combined treatments.

We used the premise of *evidence-based practice* as defined in the Institute of Medicine (2001) report: practice that "involves the integration of best research evidence with clinical expertise and patient values" (p. 145). We recognize this is a narrow definition of evidence-based practice but consider it necessary to meet the charge of conducting a consistent, comparative analysis of psychotropic medications relative to psychosocial interventions.

This is in concert with the American Psychological Association (APA; 2005) *Policy Statement on Evidence-Based Practice in Psychology*. We relied on and report the best available evidence for each major class of child and adolescent disorder. We acknowledge and advise readers that the strength of available evidence is variable across disorders. We also advise readers that for some disorders the samples enrolled in clinical trials are not necessarily representative of the children and adolescents seen in usual care settings, in which factors such as gender differences, race and ethnicity, socioeconomic status, sexual orientation, and co-occurring disorders are often present.

In preparing this book, we reviewed literature in peer-reviewed journals (included as part of Medline and PsycINFO). Available FDA data on safety were closely examined. This review was organized in accord with the nosology in the *Diagnostic and Statistical Manual of Mental Disorders* (4th ed., text rev.; *DSM–IV–TR*; American Psychiatric Association, 2000). Accurate definitions and strong methodologies are paramount to the evaluation of potential benefit (efficacy and effectiveness) and potential harm (safety) of the treatments reviewed. The conceptual framework considers acute, long-term, and adverse outcomes associated with various psychosocial and pharmacological interventions. The efficacy and safety of these interventions, and contextual variables that may affect their use and risk–benefit ratios, received primary emphasis. The review focuses on symptoms of disorders and functional outcomes. We rated the strength of evidence and magnitude of effect according to treatment modalities. Although careful assessment is always critical before treatment, for this book we were not charged with the tasks of assessment and diagnostic issues (for a review, see Mash & Hunsley, 2005).

In this chapter, we describe contextual factors that enrich understanding of various issues covered in the book. In subsequent chapters psychosocial, pharmacological, and combined interventions for each childhood and adolescent disorder are reviewed. Note that preschoolers are defined as children 5 years old and younger, children are defined as ages 6 through 12, and adolescents are defined as age 13 and above. Included in other chapters are discussions of strength of evidence, side effects, limitations, diversity, risk–benefit analysis, and future directions. The last chapter has recommendations for training and professional practice, further research, public education, and public policy.

EVALUATION OF BENEFIT

A treatment or combination of treatments is considered efficacious if carefully conducted scientific studies show that it has a positive effect on one or more outcomes of primary importance and interest. A more dimensional definition is that efficacy is the potency of an intervention, as assessed under highly controlled conditions (Bower, 2003). Efficacy studies are usually conducted in university or university-affiliated settings where it is possible to safeguard internal validity closely. When a promising treatment emerges, efficacy studies must be one component of the treatment development process and must occur prior to broad dissemination efforts. They may be conducted prior to, at the same time as, or in integration with effectiveness studies (discussed later in this section) that evaluate the effects of treatments under conditions approximating usual care (Wells, 1999).

Advances in evidence bases for clinical practices typically follow a progression from descriptive case reports to case series and open trials and ultimately to controlled single-subject, crossover, and between-groups trials. Several methodology features determine the scientific rigor of treatment studies and the extent to which findings provide definitive or interpretable information on the treatment's efficacy. Some of these features are subject flow (e.g., enrollment, intervention allocation, follow-up, data analysis); randomization procedures; control conditions (e.g., wait list, no treatment, placebo, active treatment); assessment procedures (e.g., independent blind evaluators); specification of treatment details (e.g., format, strength, duration, dose); issues related to treatment integrity and fidelity, which is the accuracy with which treatments are measured (e.g., highly trained providers, fidelity assessments); and data analysis strategies (e.g., intent to treat). A Consolidated Standards of Reporting Trials statement is available to assist investigators in outlining and reporting the design, conduct, analysis, and interpretation of their clinical trials (Begg et al., 1996; Moher, Schulz, & Altman, 2001). In the interpretation and reporting of findings, it is extremely important for investigators to be careful in their consideration and discussion of the potential generalizability of findings.

As discussed by Kaslow and Thompson (1998) and more recently by Weisz, Jensen Doss, and Hawley (2005), substantial methodological weaknesses exist in many child and adolescent treatment studies. In their analysis of 236 youths from psychotherapy outcome studies conducted across a 40-year period from 1962 through 2002, Weisz et al. found that inadequate sample sizes and the absence of procedures to enhance treatment measurement accuracy may have resulted in less than optimal tests of treatment efficacy in many studies. Additionally, other studies often failed to examine alternative explanations for positive findings, such as positive expectancies, therapeutic alliance, and attention (Jensen, Weersing, Hoagwood, & Goldman, 2005).

Because the research design and methodological strength of treatment studies vary enormously and yet are critical to the interpretation of findings of treatment efficacy, we include efficacy summary tables describing treatments of each type of child psychopathology. Using the guidelines put forth by J. Cohen (1988) for between-groups designs, we report the level of efficacy for each treatment according to effect sizes: a = .81+, large; b = .51 to .80, medium; c = .21 to .50, small; d = .20 or less. For other designs, appropriate effect sizes were considered. Tables also report the strength of evidence available for making this determination: 1 = replicated clinical or large-body, single-subject study; 2 = controlled clinical trial or replicated, single-subject study; 3 = comparison group but not clinical trial; 4 = no control group.

In more than 1,000 efficacy studies, researchers have demonstrated substantial benefits for psychotherapy and medication used together and delivered under structured treatment protocols and systematically controlled conditions. These findings hold true across a wide variety of child and adolescent mental health problems (Kazdin, 2000; Weisz & Jensen, 2001). Unfortunately, growing evidence suggests that outcomes for psychotherapy (e.g., Weersing & Weisz, 2002) and medication (Jensen et al., 1999; Multimodal Treatment of ADHD Cooperative Group, 1999a, 1999b) achieved in actual community settings fall far short compared with evidence-based clinical trials. Investigators found that both prospective controlled trials and meta-analytic reviews show that traditional psychotherapy delivered in actual community settings is on average no more effective than minimal or no intervention at all (Weiss, Catron, Harris, & Phung, 1999; Weisz, Donenberg, Han, & Weiss, 1995). For psychopharmacology, Jensen et al. (1999) found that prescriptions of stimulant medication by community pediatricians notably exceeded evidence-based guidelines. The frequent use of polypharmacy in the community far outstrips the few published studies that support this practice (Zonfrillo, Penn, & Henrietta, 2005). This fact that frequent polypharmacy is not supported by research but is frequently used in community settings, sometimes referred to as the efficacy-effectiveness paradox (Curry & Wells, 2005), presents a significant challenge to mental health research and treatment professionals.

A number of factors underlie the efficacy-effectiveness paradox. First, as previously noted, efficacy studies are designed to test the effect of treatment under optimal conditions (Connor-Smith & Weisz, 2003) and reflect design elements uncharacteristic of and difficult to achieve in the typical clinical practice. These may include the use of treatments specifically crafted to address a disorder, a wealth of experienced and highly trained therapists, careful monitoring of treatment, and opportunity to select highly motivated patients with fewer life and disease complications. In contrast, effectiveness studies seek to test the effect of treatments provided in real-world community settings. Factors more common to these studies include community therapists with varying levels of specialized expertise, limited oversight of treatments, and patient groups that are relatively heterogeneous with respect to clinical presentation and level of complexity (Connor-Smith & Weisz, 2003; Curry & Wells, 2005).

SAFETY, ETHICAL, AND LEGAL ISSUES

Issues of safety in treatment studies are being increasingly scrutinized, with recent directives from the U.S. Food and Drug Administration for safety outcomes to be as rigorously measured and monitored as efficacy outcomes.This is evidenced by the recent requirement of data and safety monitoring plans for all federally funded clinical trials and by heightened public awareness of safety issues (for review, see R. T. Brown & Zygmont, in press). It is our position that the highest possible safety standards should be applied to pediatric treatment studies. Ethical practice implies and requires partnership with the individual being treated. Various states have enacted statutes addressing such issues as a minor's legal right to consent to treatment, to give assent, to exercise a veto over treatment, or to otherwise have a meaningful say in treatment decision making. Concerns are especially pronounced with older children who, according to research, make medical decisions that are comparable to those made by adults (for review, see R. T. Brown, Daly, & Rickel, 2007). With children having more input into their treatment, understanding the abilities of each development stage gains considerably more importance. Consider the example of a 16-year-old who does not want the sexual side effects of a medication but whose parents want the medication administered. The situation becomes more complex when the actual patient is considered. Alternatively, consider a 14-year-old who desperately wants the medication to alleviate symptoms but whose parents do not want the medication administered because of its potential influence on pubertal development. It would seem ethically responsible to offer young patients and their parents psychoeducation explaining the numerous psychosocial and pharmacological factors and treatments. We recommend that readers acquaint themselves with ethics regulations. The APA "Ethical Principles of Psychologists and Code of Conduct" (APA, 2002) provides a comprehensive review of legal and ethical constants for psychosocial and psychopharmacological treatments.

Safety of psychotropic medications in children cannot be inferred from adult data (Vitiello, 2003). More research is necessary on numerous variables. These include child and parent motivation for research participation, effectiveness of the informed consent and assent process, the possibility of persistent consequences of exposure to experimental treatments and placebo, and validation of the concept of minimal risk.

Methodologies for assessing safety in children are being developed and redesigned to help standardize the collection of safety data (Greenhill et al., 2003). Measuring both efficacy and safety in a clinical trial has implications for study design. Larger sample sizes and longer durations may be necessary to identify potentially rare (e.g., SSRI-triggered suicidality) or slowly emerging (e.g., stimulant-induced height suppression for ADHD) problems, and there is a need to standardize the definitions of adverse events, degree of severity, ascertainment methods, and recording procedures (Vitiello et al., 2003).

Safety issues gain salience when psychotropic medication is used. Whether one subscribes to the Hippocratic dictum "first do no harm" or takes a risk–benefit approach to treatment, it is unethical to discount possible unwanted treatment effects. A perspective that asks "How many children should benefit from a psychotropic medication to justify one extra child harmed?" must be considered. This is a question behavioral and medical scientists must scrutinize, and indeed, the public is already doing so. One method for quantifying this question is calculating the numbers needed to benefit one additional child (NNTB; Sackett, Richardson, Rosemberg, & Haynes, 2000) and the numbers needed to treat to cause harm in one additional child (NNTH) to help researchers and clinicians weigh the relative costs and benefits of psychopharmacological and psychosocial interventions alone or in combination (Whittington et al., 2004).

The acceptability of the risk–benefit profile for any psychotropic medication thus involves value judgments of the cost of harm-related and psychiatric-related adverse events. For example, in the case of antidepressants, the risk of increased suicidality appears to be relatively low (i.e., 2 patients who experienced suicidal thoughts or intent for every 100 patients treated with an SSRI compared with a placebo), and no patients actually completed suicide in the FDA database of controlled trials. However, given the potentially lethal implications of suicidality, even low rates are important. Also, many investigators conducting trials have addressed monotherapy, whereas almost none have studied adverse-effects occurrence associated with combinations of psychotropic medications. This is surprising and worrisome because combined pharmacological treatments are often the norm in the community (Safer, Zito, & DosReis, 2003).

The debate over the possible link between the newer antidepressants and suicidality has focused public attention on the ethical and legal issues surrounding the provision of pediatric mental health care. These issues include the public's need for trust in the research and regulatory processes that determine the efficacy and safety of pediatric mental health treatments and the clinicians' role in providing ethical care directly to youth and their families.

Recent safety concerns about antidepressants illustrate several ethical issues related to clinical research and the dissemination of findings from clinical studies. These include potential miscoding of data, selective reporting and publication bias, lack of reliable and valid assessment of side effects, and failure to apply validated, empirical methodology to the examination of adverse events. A recent review urged caution in interpreting trials in children sponsored by the pharmaceutical industry, given evidence of selective reporting and a failure to publish negative results (T. Kendall, Pilling, & Whittington, 2005). Bias is not limited to financial conflicts of interest or research involving the pharmaceutical industry. Other influences, such as overly avid career advancement interests, professional affiliation, training and experience, theoretical orientation, and funding sources, may also result in bias (Levinsky, 2002). A collaborative agreement reached by medical journals to address the issue of publication bias now requires public registration of all clinical trials before papers can qualify for publication (DeAngelis et al., 2004). In the end, total transparency with all raw data involving human participants may become the only solution (Antonuccio, Danton, & McClanahan, 2003).

DEVELOPMENTAL AND CONTEXTUAL CONSIDERATIONS

Interventions for child and adolescent psychopathology have historically been drawn from the adult literature and adapted to meet the needs of children, with varying degrees of success (R. T. Brown & Sammons, 2002). Developmental processes are, of course, paramount in psychologists' understanding of children and adolescents. As noted by others (for reviews, see R. T. Brown & Sawyer, 1998; Werry & Aman, 1999), youths differ both qualitatively and quantitatively from adults. Developmental psychology generally suggests that there are periods during childhood and adolescence in which children evidence different cognitions and behaviors, including early childhood (i.e., infancy, toddlerhood, primary school years), middle childhood (i.e., elementary school years), preadolescence, early adolescence, and late adolescence.

Even in childhood, however, there are broad developmental differences that influence physiological, cognitive, behavioral, and affective functioning. Each of these areas of functioning varies by age and has influence on functional outcomes for children, particularly in school performance and socialization. For example, adolescents have the potential to be more active and cognitively engaged in their treatment than younger children and are apt to give better information about adverse side effects and potential benefits of medication.

Numerous pediatric psychology investigators report rather poor adherence to nonpsychiatric pharmacological treatments (e.g., antibiotics) and even worse adherence to psychotropic agents (for review, see La Greca & Bearman, 2003). This adherence rate differs across age groups, ethnic groups, and socioeconomic status. Poor adherence rates are a concern because of their likely effect on the increase or decrease of medication on the part of the provider. Issues of adherence may also result in family conflict, especially between the parent and child (La Greca & Bearman, 2003). Most studies of psychotropic agents use standards of clinical trials; however, such controlled situations are rare when children are prescribed medication in the family environment. We recommend that future studies create interventions geared to increase adherence rates in family environments in which real-world problems impede the ability to maintain adherence.

Development also has implications for medication titration and management. Physiological differences in children and adolescents across age categories affect rates of medication absorption, distribution in the body, and metabolism. These differ markedly from youths of different ages and from adults (R. T. Brown & Sammons, 2002). Children are also less likely than adults to give clear descriptions of changes in their physiological and psychological functioning that may be associated with the use of psychotropic medications. They may have difficulty charting the course of these changes over time and the adverse effects of these medications.

Another factor when treating children and adolescents with medication is that caregivers typically are responsible for both the decision to use pharmacotherapy and the administration of medication. At school, it may be the school nurse or the teacher who administers medication. As a result, caregiver and school personnel attitudes toward medication may influence children's use of medication and adherence to medical regimens. The unique issues in child and adolescent psychopharmacology must be considered when prescribing and monitoring medication effects at home and at school.

As R. T. Brown and Sawyer (1998) pointed out, it is hoped that use of psychotropic medication is only one element of a child's treatment program. Psychotropic medications are used to reduce children's symptoms and increase function. This increase in function makes children more amenable to other psychosocial, social, or educational interventions. The effects of development on participation in these additional interventions and the appropriate sequencing of psychosocial and psychotropic interventions during different developmental windows remain underresearched areas.

DIVERSITY

Gender, race, ethnicity, sexual orientation, physical disability, socioeconomic status, culture, and religious preference are some of the diversity variables that may moderate response to treatment and influence treatment choice and adherence. We reviewed numerous studies on treatment efficacy and found the paucity of data concerning these possible moderators alarming in comparison with data on treatment choice or use. Data on the interaction of these factors and the impact and effectiveness of pharmacological agents are very limited, and in most studies, participants were White boys. It is clear that researchers need to turn attention toward the ways diversity plays a widespread role in diagnosis and, worse, misdiagnosis. There is concern, for example, that ADHD is underdiagnosed in girls (for review, see Hinshaw et al., 1997). It should be no surprise that emerging research indicates that culture is a mediator in the response to psychosocial and pharmacological treatment. This area should be studied carefully, intensively, and immediately. Linguistic differences, immigrant status, lifestyle and health concerns, use of indigenous healers, and other cultural diversities are part of the context that determines the use of medication by children and adolescents. The shortage of data about these possible moderators in pediatric populations must be rectified so they will be better understood and more accurate interventions used.

Very little work has been done about differential metabolism of medications in children by gender, race, and ethnicity. One exception was a study conducted by Campbell et al. (1997) in a prospective investigation of neuroleptic-related dyskinesias in children with autism. The researchers found that dyskinesias were higher among girls than among boys. This investigation demonstrates the startling variability of gender as a risk factor for specific adverse effects associated with psychotropic agents. Researchers studying adults show differential metabolism of psychotropic medications by race and ethnicity. African Americans experience a greater frequency of toxicities associated with lithium carbonate. Taiwanese may respond more favorably to these agents (Strickland, Lin, Fu, Anderson, & Zheng, 1995; Yang, 1985). Even more compelling are data showing different rates of metabolism of antidepressant medication in Asian Americans compared with other ethnic groups. Conversely, greater toxicities have been shown in African Americans compared with Asian Americans, Latinos, and Whites (for reviews, see R. T. Brown & Sawyer, 1998; Phelps, Brown, & Power, 2002). Similar findings have been revealed for anxiolytic agents (for review, see R. T. Brown & Sammons, 2002; R. T. Brown & Zygmont, in press). These differential absorption rates, pharmacokinetics, and toxicities in adult ethnic group members only highlight the need for similar research on youth. Moderating effects of age, ethnicity, and gender have been found for a number of psychosocial interventions (e.g., Drotar, 2006). Indeed, adding developmental stage differences in youth may reveal even more effect on children than adults, and in many areas.

ASSESSMENT

Three assumptions governed our thinking about the clinical trials and data that formed the foundation for this book: (a) Psychopathology can be accurately diagnosed in children and adolescents, (b) interventions (whether psychopharmacological or behavioral) are clearly described and followed, and (c) outcomes are measured accurately. Stating that a particular intervention is likely to work for children and adolescents with a particular disorder assumes those individuals are reliably distinguishable from individuals not having that particular disorder and from individuals having other disorders. When it is declared that a particular intervention has a positive outcome (X), it is assumed that the intervention was implemented as described (Y), and that the outcome (Z; e.g., the reduction of symptoms from preintervention to postintervention) is reliably and accurately measured. Should these assumptions be invalid, it would be inaccurate and unethical to report that treatment X works for condition Y as measured by outcome Z. Unless conditions, treatments, and outcomes are measured accurately (i.e., reliably) and appropriately (i.e., validly), conclusions drawn from such outcome data are more dangerous than no data at all.

Researchers in assessment find that the intentions of diagnostic precision, intervention fidelity, and outcome accuracy are imperfectly realized (Mash & Hunsley, 2005). With respect to *DSM–IV–TR* (American Psychiatric Association, 2000) diagnoses, highly trained clinicians typically show good agreement when distinguishing psychopathology from normative behaviors (e.g., Klin, Lang, Cicchetti, & Volkmar, 2001) but show much less agreement when assigning specific diagnoses. This is also true when attempts are made to determine a primary diagnosis from multiple disorders. For example, differential diagnosis of ADHD from oppositional defiant disorder (ODD) continues to complicate diagnosis of the most common problem (i.e., ADHD) confronting children and adolescents (Barkley, 2003; Root & Resnick, 2003). Depth of information about a case may increase the confidence a clinician has in the diagnosis but not necessarily the accuracy of the diagnosis (Gutkind et al., 2001). Concerns about diagnostic accuracy are likely to overestimate the accuracy actually achieved in community practice with children and adolescents for two reasons. Researchers typically use clearly specified diagnostic protocols with trained professionals, whereas clinicians tend to rely on less structured diagnostic processes (Aegisdóttir, White, & Spengler, 2006; Garb, 2005). Second, the focus of most research has been on adults, who are typically able to provide better information to clinicians than are children and adolescents.

The degree to which a given treatment or intervention is actually implemented is also imperfect. Failure to take medication as directed is the most common problem in treatment of many psychological and medical disorders (e.g., Byrne, Regan, & Livingston, 2006), and it is difficult to assess treatment fidelity even in motivated adults (Bauman, 2000). Because many children and adolescents receive interventions from others (e.g., teachers, parents), researchers must assess the degree to which those adults adhere to intervention protocols. Unfortunately, we know from research that interventions, even when delivered by trained professionals who agree to implement them, are often delivered at unacceptably low levels of accuracy (Wickstrom, Jones, LaFleur, & Witt, 1998). Furthermore, assessments by professionals of adherence to treatment programs are often unrelated to assessments of treatment adherence by other observers (Noell et al., 2005). Therefore, conclusions about intervention efficacy must be tempered by evidence showing wide variability in intervention integrity.

The accuracy with which outcomes are measured varies in part as a function of the measure (e.g., different instruments have different reliabilities) and because different sources of information vary in judgments about the behavior and affect of children and adolescents. Differences in raters, settings, and the domain of behavior being observed can be substantial

(Achenbach, McConaughy, & Howell, 1987) and lead to markedly different conclusions about the degree to which individuals express psychopathology (Achenbach, Krukowski, Dumenci, & Ivanova, 2005). This is particularly problematic for those evaluating outcomes for children and adolescents because measures typically rely on adult observations.

Assessment research provides constraints on the degree to which researchers and clinicians can draw conclusions about what works, for whom it works, and how well it works. Although these constraints do not invalidate the evaluation of efficacy for psychotropic and other treatments used with children and adolescents, it is clear that conclusions should be tempered by an understanding of variability with respect to diagnostic accuracy, intervention fidelity, and outcome measurement. As shown in assessment research, practitioners should institute assessment practices to measure and ensure diagnostic accuracy, treatment fidelity, and outcome precision when applying research-based interventions to their clients.

SUMMARY

We focus in this book on specific mental health disorders encountered by practicing psychologists and other professionals caring for children and adolescents. The most prevalent disorders using the nomenclature in the *DSM–IV–TR* (American Psychiatric Association, 2000) are examined. For each disorder, the various psychosocial, psychotropic, and combination treatments are reviewed, including the effect of each therapy, the strength of evidence for its efficacy, and the limitations and side effects of each treatment in the short and long term. Many studies focus on symptom management and others investigate functional outcomes, but both are addressed here. Each chapter also presents this information in table form.

The book begins with ADHD because of its high prevalence and the volume of available research. Subsequent chapters include ODD and conduct disorder, Tourette's and tic disorders, obsessive–compulsive disorder, anxiety disorders, depressive disorders and suicidality, bipolar disorder, schizophrenia spectrum disorders, autism spectrum disorders and mental retardation, anorexia nervosa and bulimia nervosa, and elimination disorders.

2

ATTENTION-DEFICIT/HYPERACTIVITY DISORDER

Attention-deficit/hyperactivity disorder (ADHD) is characterized by developmentally inappropriate levels of inattention, impulsivity, overactivity, or a combination of these, resulting in chronic functional impairment (American Psychiatric Association, 2000). Approximately 5% of the school-age children in the United States can be diagnosed with this disorder, with boy-to-girl ratios ranging between 2:1 and 6:1 (Biederman, Lopez, Boellner, & Chandler, 2002). ADHD typically emerges early in life and is a chronic disorder that places children and adolescents at higher than average risk for academic, behavioral, and social difficulties. Thus, treatment should begin as soon as the disorder is diagnosed, address multiple areas of functioning, and be implemented across settings and over potentially long periods.

The most widely studied treatments for ADHD include psychostimulant medication (e.g., methylphenidate), behavior modification strategies, and their combination. There is widespread agreement that pharmacological intervention with a central nervous system (CNS) stimulant (Greenhill & Ford, 2006; Spencer et al., 1996; Swanson, McBurnett, Christian, & Wigal, 1995), behavior modification (Pelham, Wheeler, & Chronis, 1998), and the combination of the two (American Academy of Pediatrics, 2001a) are short-term treatments that are evidence based. Some debate exists about the amount of evidence in support of each of these and about their relative effectiveness, but all three approaches have evidence accumulated over the past 3 decades. Other treatments such as nonstimulant medications (e.g., atomoxetine, clonidine), academic intervention, and social skills strategies also have been studied, and some evidence supports their effectiveness as well, albeit less than the three primary strategies. The evidence for these interventions is summarized in Table 2.1.

PSYCHOSOCIAL INTERVENTIONS

The only psychosocial treatments that have evidence of effectiveness with ADHD are behavioral interventions. Thus, we will not discuss some of the interventions that are widely used in practice (e.g., play therapy, individual counseling, neural therapy, sensory integration) but have no scientific support.

Behavior Therapy

Since the 1970s, a large number of studies have shown that behavioral interventions result in short-term amelioration of ADHD symptoms and impairment that is comparable in most domains to that obtained with low-to-moderate doses of stimulant medication (Pelham & Waschbusch, 1999). In contrast to studies of stimulant medication, which focus on improving the core symptoms of ADHD, studies of behavioral treatments have focused on improving the key areas of impairment associated with ADHD considered to mediate long-term outcomes. These include parenting practices, peer relationships, and academic and school functioning (Pelham, Fabiano, & Massetti, 2005). Behavioral treatments and studies have involved parent training in behavioral methods (Anastopoulos, Shelton, & Barkley, 2005), behavioral and academic classroom interventions (DuPaul & Stoner, 2003), interventions for problems with peers (Mrug, Hoza, & Gerdes, 2001), and often two or three of these components at the same time. It is interesting to note that studies of behavioral treatment have shown beneficial effects from preschool to adolescence (Evans, Pelham, & Grudberg, 1995; Pisterman et al., 1989). At the same time, most of the literature is on elementary school age children. Much more research with adolescents is needed (B. H. Smith, Waschbusch, Willoughby, & Evans, 2000).

Parent Training

Parent training in behavioral methods typically consists of 8 to 12 group or individual sessions to improve parenting skills, children's behavior in key domains at home (e.g., compliance with parental requests, rule-following, decreased defiant and aggressive behavior), and knowledge about the disorder (Anastopoulos, Shelton, DuPaul, & Guevremont, 1993). Studies have most often lasted a matter of months, with effects usually measured at treatment termination and again for follow-up periods of a few months. The magnitude of effects is typically moderate to large, with within-subject designs yielding larger effects than between-groups designs (Pelham & Fabiano, in press; Pelham et al., 1998). Effects are larger on the key domains of impaired functioning previously noted than they are on the *Diagnostic and Statistical Manual of Mental Disorders* (4th ed., text rev.; *DSM–IV–TR*; American Psychiatric Association, 2000) symptoms of ADHD (e.g., Multimodal Treatment of ADHD [MTA] Cooperative Group, 1999a, 2004b). Positive effects are found regardless of comorbidity, and in some studies the impact of parent training is greatest when comorbidities are present (Hartman, Stage, & Webster-Stratton, 2003; Jensen et al., 2001; Lundahl, Risser, & Lovejoy, 2006). Training parents in behavioral methods for more effective parenting is the best validated intervention for children with aggression and conduct problems (Brestan & Eyberg, 1998). This is important information because, by far, most children with conduct problems also have ADHD, and parent training effects are at least as large if not larger for children with ADHD and comorbid conduct disorder (CD) than for children with CD alone (Bor, Sanders, & Markie-Dadds, 2002; Lundahl et al., 2006). Behavioral parent training with comorbid aggressive ADHD children is one of the most well-validated interventions in the field of child therapy. Although most studies have focused on children between ages 6 and 12, investigators found similar changes in younger children (e.g., Bor et al., 2002; Pisterman et al., 1989; Sonuga-Barke, Daley, Thompson, Laver-Bradbury, & Weeks, 2001) and adolescents (Barkley, Edwards, Laneri, Fletcher, & Metevia, 2001).

Classroom Interventions

Behavioral classroom interventions for ADHD have also been widely studied over the past 3 decades (K. D. O'Leary, Pelham, Rosenbaum, & Price, 1976), are widely used in schools (Walker, Ramsey, & Gresham, 2003–2004), and are solidly evidence based (DuPaul & Eckert, 1997; Pelham & Fabiano, in press; Pelham et al., 1998). There are many different types of classroom interventions for ADHD (DuPaul & Stoner, 2003), ranging from daily report cards (DRC) to point and token systems. Programs include focus on individuals, classrooms, and school systems. As with studies of parent training, dozens of intervention studies have examined ADHD symptoms and associated functional difficulties (e.g., following classroom rules, disruptive behavior, compliance with teacher requests, getting along with classmates). Most of the studies have investigated relatively intensive programs (e.g., point system and timeout) in special education classes (A. J. Abramowitz, Eckstrand,

TABLE 2.1
Treatment Efficacy for Attention-Deficit/Hyperactivity Disorder

Treatment	Acute		Long term[a]		Side effects[b]
	Strength of evidence and effect size, Primary symptoms	Strength of evidence and effect size, Functional outcomes	Strength of evidence and effect size, Primary symptoms	Strength of evidence and effect size, Functional outcomes	
Medication					
Stimulants	1b, Impulsiveness, hyperactivity	1b, Classroom task completion, disruptive behavior, noncompliance, aggression	1b, Impulsiveness, hyperactivity	1 or 2b, Disruptive behavior, aggression, noncompliance	Anorexia, insomnia, growth suppression, potential exacerbation of risk for substance abuse.
		1c, Peer interactions and social skills		1c, Peer interactions and social skills	
				1d, Academic achievement, parent–child relationships, parenting skills	
		1d, Academic achievement, parent–child relationships, parenting skills		1 or 2d, Special education placement, high school graduation, delinquency, vocational adjustment	

Tricyclics	1c, Inattention, impulsiveness, hyperactivity	3c	3c	3c	Sedation, increased appetite, risk for cardiac toxicity.
Buproprion	2c, Inattention, impulsiveness, hyperactivity	No data	No data	No data	Rash, incremental risk for seizures.
Clonidine	1c–d, Impulsiveness, hyperactivity, inattention	1d, Disruptive behavior	No data	No data	Sedation, irritability
Atomoxetine	1c, Impulsiveness, hyperactivity, inattention	1d	1a–c, Impulsiveness, hyperactivity, inattention	No data	Aggressive behavior, liver toxicity
Psychosocial	1b, Inattention, impulsivity, hyperactivity	1b, Classroom task completion, disruptive behavior, noncompliance, aggression 1b, Peer interactions and social skills 1d, Academic achievement 1b–c, Parent–child relationships 1b–c, Parenting skills	2c, Inattention, impulsivity, hyperactivity	2c, Classroom task, completion, disruptive behavior, noncompliance, aggression 2c, Peer interactions and social skills 2d, Parent–child relationships 2c, Parenting skills	None
Combination	1b, Inattention, impulsivity, hyperactivity	1b, Classroom task completion, disruptive behavior, noncompliance, aggression	2a, Inattention, impulsivity, hyperactivity	2b, Classroom task completion, disruptive behavior, noncompliance, aggression	Same as medications alone but reduced in magnitude because doses are lower.

(continues)

TABLE 2.1
(Continued)

Treatment	Acute		Long term[a]		Side effects[b]
	Strength of evidence and effect size, Primary symptoms	Strength of evidence and effect size, Functional outcomes	Strength of evidence and effect size, Primary symptoms	Strength of evidence and effect size, Functional outcomes	
		1b, Peer interactions and social skills		2b, Peer interactions and social skills	
		1d, Academic achievement		2d, Academic achievement	
		1b, Parent–child relationships		2b, Parent–child relationships	
		1b, Parenting skills		2b, Parenting skills	

Note. Across all treatment studies for each type of child psychopathology, we used guidelines put forth by J. Cohen (1988): Strength of evidence: 1 = replicated clinical trial or large-body, single-subject study; 2 = controlled clinical trial or replicated, single-subject study; 3 = comparison group but not clinical trial; 4 = no control group. Effect size: a = .81+, large; b = .51 to .80, medium; c = .21 to .50, small; d = .20 or less.
[a]Over 12 months. [b]See side effects and risk–benefit discussion.

O'Leary, & Dulcan, 1992; Carlson, Pelham, Milich, & Dixon, 1992; Chronis et al., 2004; Northup et al., 1999; Pelham, Burrows-MacLean, et al., 2005; Pelham et al., 1993) or less intensive programs (e.g., DRC and teacher consultation) in regular class settings (Gittelman et al., 1980; S. G. O'Leary & Pelham, 1978; Pelham et al., 1988). The effects of the interventions are typically greater with the more intensive programs in special classes, though they are substantial even with DRCs in mainstream classrooms (DuPaul & Eckert, 1997; Pelham & Fabiano, in press; Pelham et al., 1998). Effects have been shown in samples of children from ages 5 to 12 (Barkley et al., 2000).

Academic Interventions

Most of the studies of classroom interventions for ADHD have focused on deportment rather than academic outcomes. Many of the studies described in previous sections included daily seat-work productivity and accuracy as outcomes, and the effect of the classroom management programs on those variables is well established (DuPaul & Eckert, 1997; Pelham & Fabiano, in press). However, these studies focus on acute daily functioning rather than achievement measured over time. In addition, results from single-subject design studies support the short-term effects of academic intervention strategies on the behavior and academic performance of children with ADHD. Specifically, preliminary evidence supports the use of modified task demands (Zentall, 1989), providing task choices (Dunlap et al., 1994), peer tutoring (DuPaul, Ervin, Hook, & McGoey, 1998), parent tutoring (Hook & DuPaul, 1999), and computer-assisted instruction (Ota & DuPaul, 2002) in enhancing on-task behavior and, in some cases, improving achievement.

Academic strategies may lead to behavior change that is equivalent in magnitude to contingency management interventions (DuPaul & Eckert, 1997) and are arguably necessary to improve academic achievement. Interventions focused on academic-related behaviors (e.g., taking notes on classroom lectures) also may benefit adolescents (Evans et al., 1995) and younger elementary school age children with ADHD (DuPaul et al., 2005). Beyond the utility of contingency management to improve daily seat-work productivity and accuracy, generalizations about the efficacy of academic interventions for these students must be tempered with findings from single-subject design studies that have been extended to larger samples in the context of controlled experimental trials and academic achievement used as an outcome.

Peer Interventions

Interventions focused on peer relationships have been less well studied compared with parent training and classroom interventions. These interventions teach social skills, social problem solving, and behavioral competencies (e.g., sports skills) while decreasing aggression and other undesirable behaviors (e.g., bossiness). They are usually provided in clinic- or school-based weekly social skills groups, after-school or weekend groups (e.g., Frankel, Myatt, Cantwell, & Feinberg, 1997), and summer camp settings (e.g., Pelham, Fabiano, Gnagy, et al., 2005). Typically, these programs are not stand-alone but integrate parent training (Pfiffner & McBurnett, 1997), school-based interventions (Pelham et al., 1988), or both (Pelham, Fabiano, Gnagy, et al., 2005).

Preliminary evidence is that weekly social skills groups might add incrementally to the effects of school-based and home-based interventions (Pfiffner & McBurnett, 1997). There is considerable evidence that an intensive program package delivered in a summer camp and including social skills training, a reward-and-cost system, group practice, and instruction in sports skills and team membership can reliably produce medium to large immediate and short-term effects (Chronis et al., 2004; Pelham, Burrows-MacLean, et al., 2005, 2007; Pelham, Gnagy, et al., 2007; Pelham & Hoza, 1996). The MTA study involved parent training, teacher consultation, and a summer camp focused on peer interventions (Wells, Pelham, et al., 2000). The interventions resulted in large pre–post-improvements that maintained at 1- and 2-year follow-up (MTA Cooperative Group, 1999a, 2004a, 2004b). Studies of these intensive summer interventions have included children ranging from 5 to 14 years of age.

Strength of Evidence

Numerous studies summarized in several reviews have shown that effect sizes for psychosocial interventions are in the moderate-to-large range, depending on the type of study design. DuPaul and Eckert (1997) and Pelham and Fabiano (in press) concluded that the mean effect size in between-groups behavioral studies was between .5 and .7 (see also Lundahl et al., 2006). DuPaul and Eckert's meta-analysis focused on school-based studies, Lundahl et al. focused on parent training, and Pelham and Fabiano examined studies across settings, including home, school, peer, and recreation. Effect sizes in crossover designs are computed with a different metric and are rarely included in traditional meta-analyses. When analyzed, they reveal a large effect by behavioral treatment, yielding considerably larger effect sizes compared with between-groups studies. Effect sizes in studies with single-subject designs are even larger in meta-analyses that have included them.

As discussed later in this chapter, all of these effects are in the same range as those that have been summarized in reviews of stimulant medication. The only review that has separated the effects of behavior modification by domain (Fabiano, Pelham, Coles, et al., 2007) has shown that these effect sizes are consistent across multiple functional domains, behaviors, and assessment methods. When academic achievement has been assessed, few studies have lasted long enough to measure achievement. As with medication, behavioral treatments have had little effect on long-term academic achievement. When acute measures of academic functioning are assessed, effect sizes are in the moderate-to-large range for seat-work productivity but in the small range for achievement measures.

Limitations

Although there is considerable evidence for effective behavioral interventions for ADHD in children and adolescents, there are some limitations. Chief among these are that behavioral treatments (a) do not work to the same degree for all children and are not sufficient for some, (b) can be relatively more expensive than medication alone in the short run, (c) have far more evidence for acute than for long-term effects, and (d) must be simultaneously implemented across settings and domain (i.e., parent training, school interventions, and peer interventions need to be done conjointly to affect all three domains). The first, third, and fourth of these limitations also apply to stimulant medications (see discussion in the next section). Given that both stimulant medications and behavioral treatments have limitations, many professionals believe that combined interventions are most effective and should be used routinely.

PHARMACOLOGICAL INTERVENTIONS

The most widely used interventions for ADHD in the mental health field are pharmacotherapeutic approaches. CNS stimulants have been used for ADHD for more than 50 years, while the other medications described in the following sections are mostly nonapproved for ADHD, are used far less often, and are far less effective.

Stimulants

CNS stimulant compounds (e.g., methylphenidate, dextroamphetamine, and mixed amphetamine salts) remain the first-choice medications for treatment of ADHD symptoms in children and adolescents (American Academy of Child & Adolescent Psychiatry, 2002; American Academy of Pediatrics, 2001b). Approximately 1.5 million children (or more than 4% of school-age children) are treated with CNS stimulants in the United States (Safer & Zito, 2000). Stimulant medication use has grown steadily throughout the past 2 decades, particularly among preschool and secondary school children (Olfson, Marcus, Weissman, & Jensen, 2002; Robison, Sclar, Skaer, & Galin, 2004). The average duration of medication use is between 2 and 7 years depending on the age of the child (Safer & Zito, 2000).

Approximately 75% of elementary school age children with ADHD treated with stimulant medications respond positively to one or more doses (e.g., Rapport & Denney, 2000). Numerous empirical studies have documented the short-term behavioral effects of stimulants, including improvements in attention and task completion, with concomitant reductions in impulsivity, disruptive behavior, and, in some cases, aggression (e.g., Greenhill et al., 2006; MTA Cooperative Group, 1999a). Similar behavioral effects have been obtained for adolescents with ADHD; however, the percentage of positive responders is lower than among elementary school children (50% compared with 70%, respectively; Evans et al., 2001; Pelham, Vodde-Hamilton, Murphy, Greenstein, & Vallano, 1991; B. H. Smith et al., 1998), especially when measured in home and school settings. Several studies also have documented stimulant-induced, short-term improvements in impulsivity, disruptive behavior, and attention among preschoolers at risk for ADHD (Barkley, 1988; Chacko et al., 2005). However, young children may be at greater risk for adverse side effects of this treatment (see Side Effects section later in this chapter). Stimulants have no effect on academic achievement in the short term, and no long-term effects have been reliably reported.

Nonstimulants

Atomoxetine is a nonstimulant compound that affects norepinephrine. In several controlled trials, this drug reduced ADHD symptoms (Michelson et al., 2001). However, the number of studies is small, and the dependent measure assessed has typically been parent or clinician symptom ratings, thus a large range of objective measures, child ratings, and more studies of stimulant effects are needed. The approved label for atomoxetine has recently been modified with warnings of potential drug-related problems in aggressive behavior, suicidality, and liver toxicity (U.S. Food and Drug Administration, 2005), although some have disputed these warnings (Barkley & Fischer, 2005). These nonstimulant compounds do not appear to be as effective as stimulants, and they have comparable (or higher) risk of side effects and are, therefore, considered second-choice pharmacological treatments (Wigal et al., 2005).

Other nonstimulant compounds evaluated as treatments for ADHD include clonidine, an antihypertensive agent. It is moderately effective in reducing ADHD symptoms (Connor, Fletcher, & Swanson, 1999) and may ameliorate sleep disturbance associated with the disorder (Prince, Wilens, Biederman, Spencer, & Wozniak, 1996). Guanfacine is an antihypertensive agent that appears to have similar behavioral effects to clonidine but has not been evaluated extensively with controlled trials (Cohn & Caliendo, 1997).

Antidepressants

Antidepressant medications, including tricyclics (Spencer, Biederman, & Wilens, 1998; Spencer, Biederman, Wilens, Steingard, & Geist, 1993) and bupropion (Casat, Pleasants, Schroeder, & Parker, 1989; Conners et al.,

1996), have been well researched. In general, antidepressants are less effective than stimulants, not FDA-approved for treatment of ADHD, and thus are considered second-line treatments, at best, for this disorder.

Combination

There is an increasing trend for CNS stimulants to be prescribed in combination with other psychotropic medications (Guevara, Lozano, Wickizer, Mell, & Gephart, 2002), presumably to counteract stimulant side effects and to address comorbid disorders. For example, the combination of clonidine and a stimulant is associated with reduced aggression and conduct problems in children with comorbid ADHD and oppositional defiant disorder (ODD) and CD (Hazell & Stuart, 2003) and with comorbid ADHD and Tourette's disorder (Kurlan et al., 2002). However, the combination was not more effective than methylphenidate alone on ADHD symptoms in school, and the combination was much less tolerable than methylphenidate or clonidine alone (Palumbo et al., 2005). Although T. E. Brown (2004) suggested that the combination of atomoxetine and a stimulant also may lead to better symptomatic improvement in children resistant to monotherapy, this combination has not been investigated in any controlled trial to date. Further, there are no safety data on this combination of medications. There are scant data on polypharmacy with these children in general, despite its widespread use.

Although they are clearly efficacious in the short term, medications have limitations. Primary among them is the lack of long-term evidence that the medications are safe when taken over a period of years (National Institutes of Health [NIH] Consensus Statement, 1998). For all nonstimulant medications, short-term safety data are also lacking. Second, there is no evidence that stimulants produce long-term benefits because long-term studies have consistently failed to provide positive evidence (MTA Cooperative Group, 2004a, 2004b, 2007; NIH Consensus Statement, 1998; Volkow & Insel, 2003). In addition, as with behavior therapy, stimulants do not normalize functioning in most children even acutely (e.g., Swanson et al., 2001). Although it is clear that stimulants improve ADHD symptoms, it is less clear that they improve functioning in key domains that are thought to mediate long-term outcomes (e.g., academic functioning, parenting skills, peer relationships).

Strength of Evidence

For the stimulants (primarily methylphenidate), effect sizes for ADHD symptoms based on ratings and observations of the adults in the child's life are in the moderate-to-large range (Conners, 2002). Effect sizes for measures of academic productivity are low to moderate, and for academic achievement they are around zero. The overall effect size for stimulant treatment is in the moderate range, with larger effects associated with teacher and parent ratings than for direct observations and lab measures. Effect sizes for atomoxetine are in the moderate-to-large range on parent and clinician symptom ratings, and the magnitude of effects for other medications (e.g., antidepressants) typically are lower than for stimulants and in the low-to-moderate range overall.

Side Effects

Potential adverse side effects of stimulants include insomnia, appetite reduction, and irritability (Connor, 2005b). Growth suppression (approximately 1 centimeter per year) has occurred with continued use over several years (MTA Cooperative Group, 2004a, 2007; Swanson et al., 2007). Growth reductions appear to be worse in young children with ADHD—approximately 1.4 centimeter per year or a 20% reduction in growth rate for both height and weight. Acute adverse side effects typically diminish with a reduction in dosage. Growth suppression can be attenuated with twice-daily versus three-times-a-day dosing and drug holidays during summer and school vacations (Connor, 2005b). Stimulant medications do not appear to exacerbate tic disorders (Gadow, Sverd, Sprafkin, Nolan, & Ezor, 1995; Kurlan et al., 2002; Palumbo, Spencer, Lynch, Co-Chien, & Faraone, 2004). Findings have been equivocal with respect to risks for substance abuse when stimulant medications are used. Approximately equal numbers of studies show no, heightened, and reduced risk (S. L. Anderson, Arvanitogiannis, Pliakas, LeBlanc, & Carlezon, 2002; Barkley, Fischer, Smallish, & Fletcher, 2003; Biederman, Wilens, Mick, Spencer, & Faraone, 1999; Pelham, Molina, Gnagy, Meichenbaum, & Greenhouse, 2007).

Nonstimulant compounds also are associated with adverse side effects. For example, atomoxetine can lead to stomachaches, nausea, decreased appetite, and failure to gain weight (Christman, Fermo, & Markowitz, 2004). As noted previously, the FDA issued a warning that atomoxetine may increase the risk of suicidal thinking in children and adolescents with ADHD; this risk is approximately 0.4% (U.S. Food and Drug Administration, 2005). Possible side effects associated with combined medication protocols have not been investigated extensively. However, most side effects of stimulants are dose related. Many studies have shown that beneficial stimulant effects are maximized at much lower doses when used in conjunction with behavioral treatment (e.g., Carlson et al., 1992; Fabiano et al., in press; Pelham, Burrows-MacLean, et al., 2005, 2007; Pelham et al., 1993; Pelham, Gnagy, et al., 2007), with a resultant benefit of combined treatments of lowered risk for such common and dose-related side effects as growth suppression.

COMBINED INTERVENTIONS

Studies of combined interventions have the same characteristics as those that have evaluated behavior therapy alone. They have been conducted in controlled settings like summer treatment programs and special classrooms (A. J. Abramowitz et al., 1992; Carlson et al., 1992; Pelham, Burrows-MacLean, et al., 2005; Pelham et al., 1993) and in regular classrooms and homes (Klein & Abikoff, 1997; MTA Cooperative Group, 1999a; Pelham et al., 1988; Pelham, Schnedler, Bologna, & Contreras, 1980). In a prototypic finding in a controlled setting, Carlson et al. (1992) reported that the effects of a behavioral intervention and 0.3 milligram/kilogram of methylphenidate were equivalent and additive on several measures of behavior, such that the combination of the two resulted in behavioral improvement equal to the 0.6-milligram/kilogram dose of methylphenidate alone.

Pelham, Burrows-MacLean, et al. (2005; also Fabiano et al., in press; Pelham, Burrows-MacLean, et al., 2007; Pelham, Gnagy, et al., 2007) recently extended this finding by reducing the dose to 0.15 milligram/kilogram, indicating that very low doses of a stimulant plus a behavioral intervention maximize efficacy in a combined treatment regimen. In these studies, the 0.15-milligram/kilogram regimen produced no side effects. As noted previously, this is one of the major benefits of combined interventions for ADHD—better acute efficacy with lower doses and lower side effects. It is interesting to note that when high-intensity doses of either medication or behavior therapy are used, little evidence appears for the value of combined interventions (Abikoff et al., 2004; Pelham et al., 2000). This makes sense statistically given that a high dose of one effective treatment, regardless of treatment type or modality, often leaves little room for improvement with an additional intervention.

The between-groups studies in natural settings also show evidence of combined treatment effects, but there are fewer studies, and the effects are somewhat smaller than in controlled settings compared with medication alone. For example, in the MTA Cooperative Group (1999a) study, all four treatment groups—study medication, community treatment (mostly medicated by community physicians), behavior therapy, and combined interventions—showed large improvements from baseline to end of treatment, with relatively small differences among them. Further, secondary analyses showed clearly that combined treatment was superior to medication alone on almost every dependent measure. Combined treatments were better for comorbid children, impairments in multiple domains (vs. *DSM–IV–TR* symptoms of ADHD), parent–child relations, normalization, and consumer satisfaction with treatment (Conners et al., 2001; Jensen et al., 2001; MTA Cooperative Group, 1999b; Pelham, Erhardt, et al., 2007; Swanson et al., 2001; Wells, Epstein, et al., 2000; Wells et al., 2006). It is interesting to note that at 10-

month follow-up, the combined treatment group was superior to the group with behavior therapy only on ADHD and ODD symptoms and not on any other domain of functioning (e.g., social skills, parent–child relationships, academic achievement). This was accounted for because 50% of the apparent incremental value of the medication component of the combined treatment condition had been lost, in part because some participants stopped taking medication, whereas the effects of the behavioral intervention had completely maintained, with only a minority having initiated pharmacotherapy (MTA Cooperative Group, 2004a, 2004b). Another 50% of the medication effect was lost with 1 more year of follow-up, leaving the combined group no different from the behavioral treatment and the medication groups (MTA Cooperative Group, 2007). This outcome is consistent with earlier, smaller studies (Gittelman et al., 1980; Pelham et al., 1988) that showed when medication is withdrawn from a combined regimen, the medication effect is lost but the behavioral effect is maintained.

Strength of Evidence

Effect sizes associated with combined stimulant–behavioral interventions are about the same as for stimulants alone (moderate-to-large) when impact on ADHD symptoms are examined (MTA Cooperative Group, 1999a). Alternatively, except when ceiling effects are present, combined stimulant–behavioral treatment protocols lead to larger effects (in the moderate-to-large range) than for medication alone for a wide range of associated difficulties, such as conduct problems, oppositional behavior, social skills, and disruptive behaviors in classroom, home, and recreational and peer settings (Carlson et al., 1992; Conners et al., 2001; Fabiano et al., in press; Jensen et al., 2001; MTA Cooperative Group, 1999b; Pelham, Burrows-MacLean, et al., 2005, 2007; Pelham et al., 1993; Pelham, Gnagy, et al., 2007; Swanson et al., 2001; Wells, Epstein, et al., 2000; Wells et al., 2006). Combined treatment effects are in the moderate range for daily measures of academic seat-work productivity (e.g., Carlson et al., 1992; Fabiano et al., in press; Pelham, Burrows-MacLean, et al., 2005). As would be expected given the lack of evidence for benefit on long-term achievement of either of the two components alone, there is no evidence so far of combined treatment effects on academic achievement.

Limitations

The primary advantage of combined behavioral and stimulant interventions for ADHD is that they address the limitations of each of the separate interventions, as previously discussed, and thus have relatively fewer limitations. The limitations would be the same as those listed for the separate components. One additional limitation is that there is less evidence for the combined approach than for either component alone, especially in the long term.

DIVERSITY

Although the most common treatments for ADHD are stimulant medication (42%) and psychosocial interventions (32%), patterns of use and treatment response may vary as a function of such demographic factors as gender, ethnicity, and age (Robison et al., 2004). Most investigations of treatment outcome in ADHD have focused on elementary school age White boys from middle-class backgrounds. Although research on girls with ADHD has increased in recent years, only a few studies of gender differences in treatment response are available, and those indicate comparable responsiveness across genders (e.g., Pelham, Walker, Sturges, & Hoza, 1989). The MTA Cooperative Group (1999a, 1999b) study did not find gender to be a significant predictor of treatment outcome. Researchers and practitioners alike, however, should take note that data from at least two studies showed that girls with ADHD are less likely to be treated for their symptoms, particularly with stimulant medication, than boys with this disorder (Bussing et al., 2005; Robison et al., 2004).

There may be important differences in treatment acceptability and response between racial and ethnic groups, especially in relation to the use of stimulant medication. For example, African American children may experience higher blood pressure with stimulant treatment (R. T. Brown & Sexson, 1987). Several investigators suggest a lower use of psychotropic medication as a treatment for ADHD for African Americans (Stevens, Harman, & Kelleher, 2005) and that higher dosages of stimulants are used with White children (Lipkin, Cozen, Thompson, & Mostofsky, 2005). African American children with ADHD may be more likely to receive special education services than non-African American children with this disorder (Bussing et al., 2005). This differential treatment may be related to racial differences in acceptability of pharmacological treatment approaches, disparities in insurance coverage as a function of socioeconomic status, or lack of awareness and practice differences on the part of mostly White practitioners. The MTA Cooperative Group suggested a greater need for and response to multimodal treatment on some measures among non-White children with ADHD relative to their White peers (A. L. Arnold et al., 2003). On other measures (e.g., improvement in referred problems, parent satisfaction), treatment effects were independent of ethnicity (Pelham, Erhardt, et al., 2007; Pelham & Hoza, 1996).

As discussed earlier, developmental factors may also play a role in treatment. For example, total daily dosages of stimulants (Lipkin et al., 2005) and the use of combined treatment protocols (Robison et al., 2004) increase with age. In recent years, the largest increases in stimulant use are found among adolescents in the 12- to 18-year-old age range (Olfson, Gameroff, Marcus, & Jensen, 2003). Further research examining treatment effects and outcomes by diversity variables is necessary.

RISK–BENEFIT ANALYSIS

The most important consideration in treatment for children with ADHD is an analysis of the risks and benefits associated with the two treatment modalities and whether the relative benefits outweigh the relative risks. Behavioral treatments, pharmacotherapy with CNS stimulants, and combined behavioral and stimulant interventions are all solid evidence-based, short-term treatments for ADHD. With medium effect sizes, they improve ADHD symptoms and associated impairments, with stimulants having a larger effect on the former and behavioral treatments on the latter. Both forms of treatment have limitations that are addressed in part by combination therapies, giving rise to the popularity of multimodal treatments. Given that the acute side effects of stimulants are relatively minor and can be controlled by reducing dose or stopping medication, the risk–benefit analysis of the acute effects of stimulants is very favorable. The same is true for behavioral treatments, which have no known risks. Although some have argued that the rewards that are integral to behavior modification may have an iatrogenic effect on intrinsic motivation (Akin-Little, Eckert, Lovett, & Little, 2004), careful analysis of this issue fails to support this notion (also see discussion that follows regarding deviancy treatment in group settings). Because combined treatments yield relatively larger effects with relatively lower doses of medication, a risk–benefit analysis of them compared with medication alone would be favorable because they produce larger effects with fewer side effects.

Despite the evidence that they are effective in the short term, there is little evidence documenting long-term effects of any intervention for ADHD, and the risk–benefit analysis is different for long-term use of medication. There is no evidence that stimulants produce effects that maintain over years, generalize after medication is stopped, or alter long-term outcomes of treated individuals. A growing concern is that growth suppression will almost always occur with long-term use of stimulants. As discussed previously, there is not enough clarity about the long-term risks of stimulants in other domains (e.g., potential elevation of risk for substance use). With use beyond 2 to 3 years, the risk–benefit analysis of stimulant medication does not appear to be favorable because beneficial effects seem to dissipate and side effects do not. The long-term risk–benefit ratio of stimulants (e.g., adult outcomes) is not known because even though there are not apparent long-term benefits, long-term side effects have not been studied.

Only one study focused on the long-term use of behavioral treatment, and that study (MTA Cooperative Group, 1999a, 2004b) showed that the acute benefits of behavioral treatments maintained over time (up to 2 years posttreatment). Thus, at least in this instance, the risk–benefit ratio of behavioral treatment over a fairly extended time was favorable. There are no studies of behavioral treatment into adulthood, and the risk–benefit ratio is not known. The MTA is also the only study of longer term effects of combined treatment. At the 2-year follow-up, children in combined treatment had the same outcomes as those in behavioral treatment alone, and they had growth suppression just as the medication-alone children did. Growth suppression, however, was less in this cohort because of lower dosages. In general, the use of combined treatments for 2 to 3 years would not appear to have a favorable risk–benefit ratio. There are no studies of combined treatment into adulthood.

For this regimen to have a favorable risk–benefit ratio, there would need to be incrementally beneficial improvements relative to behavioral treatment alone without a corresponding increase in side effects. There is some indication from one short-term study that such an outcome might be attainable with very low dosages of stimulants (Fabiano et al., in press; Pelham, Burrows-MacLean, et al., 2007; Pelham, Gnagy, et al., 2007), but more research is needed.

Despite widespread use, other interventions (e.g., neural feedback, cognitive behavior therapy, antidepressants) have little or no evidence base of support, so a risk–benefit analysis would not be considered favorable. This would be particularly true for antidepressants, which have lower efficacy and higher side effects compared with stimulants.

FUTURE DIRECTIONS

One issue that has not been researched despite its importance in clinical practice is the sequence in which interventions should be implemented for treating ADHD. Should medication be used as the first-line treatment, which is the most common practice and the preference of many, if not most, physicians? If so, how long should it be tried and at what doses before, and if, behavioral interventions are added? Alternatively, should behavior modification be implemented first, and if so, how should the components (i.e., parent training, school intervention, and peer intervention) be sequenced? How long should behavior modification be tried and at what intensity before medication is added? Might a behavioral-treatment-first sequence result in less use of stimulants or lower doses with fewer side effects? Or should the two major modalities begin simultaneously so that all children receive both modalities?

Given that ADHD is recognized as a chronic disorder and treatment needs to be implemented over long periods, a relevant question is when can treatment be stopped? Which components can be time limited, and how does treatment need to be modified as children move through different developmental stages? Given the minimal effect of medication and psychosocial interventions on academic achievement, particularly over the long term, what academic interventions are efficacious with children and adolescents diagnosed with ADHD? How can these and other behavioral treatments be delivered feasibly in schools? These are questions that beg answers, and more questions exist. Studies must directly and systematically investigate these issues.

3

OPPOSITIONAL DEFIANT AND CONDUCT DISORDERS

Children and adolescents with *oppositional defiant disorder* (ODD) have high levels of noncompliance, defiance, and disruptive behavior (American Psychiatric Association, 2000). *Conduct disorder* (CD), a more serious disruptive behavior disorder, includes violation of major norms and rules of society (e.g., stealing) as well as covert or overt antisocial behavior. Approximately 2% to 16% of children in the United States have ODD and 1% to 10% have CD, with boys at higher risk for both diagnoses. ODD typically begins early in life and can be chronic through adolescence. There are two forms of CD, one beginning in childhood and the other beginning in adolescence. Childhood-onset CD is more serious in terms of severity and chronicity of antisocial behavior (Moffitt, Caspi, Dickson, Silva, & Stanton, 1996). Children and adolescents with ODD or CD are at higher-than-average risk for attention-deficit/hyperactivity disorder (ADHD), family and social relationship difficulties, academic underachievement, delinquency, and eventual prison placement as adults (Frick & Loney, 1999).

PSYCHOSOCIAL INTERVENTIONS

Psychosocial interventions, the most widely studied treatment approach for children with ODD and CD, include home-based behavior modification

(Webster-Stratton, 1994), school-based behavior modification (Walker, Colvin, & Ramsey, 1995), cognitive behavior therapy (Lochman & Wells, 2004), combined intervention approaches (Kazdin, Seigel, & Bass, 1992), and residential treatment (Chamberlain, Fisher, & Moore, 2002).

With home-based behavior modification, parents typically receive training in antecedent-based (e.g., giving effective commands) and consequent-based (e.g., token reinforcement, response cost, and timeout from positive reinforcement) interventions that usually target child compliance and task completion. In a similar fashion, school-based behavior modification approaches include the use of contingent teacher praise or reprimands, token reinforcement, response cost, timeout from positive reinforcement, and self-management (e.g., self-monitoring, self-reinforcement). Most school-based interventions are implemented directly by teachers; however, contingencies can also be delivered by peers (Cunningham & Cunningham, 1998) or parents (e.g., Pelham et al., 1993).

Home- and school-based contingency management interventions are associated with significant improvements in compliance and concomitant reductions in aggression and disruptive behavior with children (Walker et al., 1995; Webster-Stratton, 1994), but these effects are less pronounced in adolescents. Generalization of effects across settings and time is limited. Behavioral parent training is associated with a medium effect size for reduction of externalizing behaviors (Maughan, Christiansen, Jenson, Olympia, & Clark, 2005).

Cognitive behavior therapy (e.g., Lochman & Wells, 2004), multisystemic family treatment (Henggeler, Schoenwald, Rowland, & Cunningham, 2002), and combined contingency management and cognitive behavior therapy (e.g., Kazdin et al., 1992) have also led to reductions in covert delinquent behavior, aggression, and possibly substance use. Multisystemic treatment provides problem-focused treatment within families and also supports family members in managing the interconnected systems of family, peer, neighborhood, and school to reduce risks (e.g., interactions with antisocial peers and problematic school performance) associated with delinquency (Tolan & Gorman-Smith, 1997). Various forms of residential treatment have been studied with multidimensional-treatment foster care (Chamberlain et al., 2002) and the family teaching model (Friman et al., 1996) and have improved academic functioning and reduced arrests, incarceration, and drug use. Table 3.1 provides a summary of treatment efficacy for ODD and CD.

Strength of Evidence

Contingency management interventions implemented at home and school have resulted in moderate to large effect sizes for reduction in conduct problems (DuPaul & Eckert, 1997; Maughan et al., 2005). Cognitive behavior therapy and multisystemic therapy have also resulted in moderate effect sizes (Brestan & Eyberg, 1998). Thus, psychosocial interventions for the treatment of ODD (primarily contingency management at home and school) and CD (contingency management, cognitive behavior therapy, combined or multisystemic therapy, and, possibly, residential treatment) are supported by current research.

Limitations

Although behavioral interventions are effective for reducing symptoms of ODD and CD, these treatments have several limitations, including the following: Effects vary across children and may not be sufficient, costs can be relatively high in terms of resources and time, minimal evidence exists for long-term effects, and simultaneous implementation across settings and domain is necessary to achieve optimal effects (Fabiano & Pelham, 2002). Perhaps because behavioral strategies require consistent implementation across time and caregivers, treatment adherence rates typically are under 50% unless ongoing feedback is provided to the adult implementing the treatment (Sterling-Turner, Watson, & Moore, 2002).

PHARMACOLOGICAL INTERVENTIONS

A variety of psychotropic medications have been used to manage aggression and mood disturbance associated with CD. Although psychostimulants are not thought of as treatment for aggression in the context of disruptive behavior disorders, there are several modest-sized studies attesting to a moderate effect in some children (Aman & Lindsay, 2002). The most elaborate of these showed a sizable effect in children having CDs with and without ADHD (Klein, Abikoff, Ganeles, Seese, & Pollack, 1997). Several moderate-sized controlled trials found that lithium reduced aggressive behavior in children and adolescents with CD (Gerardin, Cohen, Mazet, & Flament, 2002; Malone, Delaney, Leubbert, Cater, & Campbell, 2000).

Controlled and open trials of classical antipsychotic medications such as haloperidol (Campbell, Cohen, & Small, 1982) found significant reductions in aggression and disruptive behavior. However, haloperidol can be associated with significant adverse side effects (e.g., significant extrapyramidal signs). Janssen Pharmaceutical launched several large-scale trials of risperidone in children with disruptive behavior disorder (DBD), either CD or ODD. Three acute trials (totaling about 250 children, mostly over a 6-week interval) found about a 50% reduction in DBD symptoms, compared with about 20% reduction with placebo (Aman & Lindsay, 2002; Findling et al., 2004; Snyder et al., 2002). Three long-term trials followed more than 600 children for 1 year, with continued suppression of DBD symptoms, but

TABLE 3.1
Treatment Efficacy for Oppositional Defiant and Conduct Disorders

Treatment	Acute		Long term[a]		
	Strength of evidence and effect size, Primary symptoms	Strength of evidence and effect size, Functional outcomes	Strength of evidence and effect size, Primary symptoms	Strength of evidence and effect size, Functional outcomes	Side effects[b]
Psychosocial					
Behavioral	1a–b, Compliance, aggression, disruptive behavior	2b, Academic functioning 3a, Peer relationships	2d, Compliance, aggression, disruptive behavior	No data	Possible social contagion effect for group treatment.
CBT	3a, Covert delinquent behavior, substance abuse	Peer relationships	2–3a, Covert delinquent behavior, substance abuse	No data	Possible social contagion effect for group treatment.
Residential	2c, Arrests, drug use	Academic functioning	No data	No data	Possible social contagion effect for group treatment.
Medication					
Lithium	2b, Aggression	No data	No data	No data	Polyuria, polydipsia, motor tremor, increased appetite, dryness of mouth, general muscular weakness, memory reduction.
Antipsychotics	2b, Aggression, disruptive behavior	No data	No data	No data	Sedation, extrapyramidal effects, headache, nausea, weight gain.

Divalproex sodium	2c, Aggression	No data	No data	No data	Abdominal pain, headache, drowsiness, dizziness, memory difficulties.
Methylphenidate and clonidine	2c, Aggression	No data	No data	No data	Sedation, appetite reduction, low blood pressure.
Atomoxetine	2a, ADHD symptoms 2b, ODD and ADHD symptoms	No data	No data	No data	Stomachaches, nausea, decreased appetite, weight loss, possible increase in suicidal thoughts.
Combination					
Methylphenidate and psychosocial for ODD and CD, with ADHD	2b, ODD and ADHD symptoms 2c, Parent–child relationships	2d, Academic functioning 2c, Peer relationships	2c, ODD and ADHD symptoms	2d, Academic functioning Peer relationships	Insomnia, appetite reduction, growth inhibition.

Note. Across all treatment studies for each type of child psychopathology, we used guidelines put forth by J. Cohen (1988): 1 = replicated clinical trial or large-body, single-subject study; 2 = controlled clinical trial or replicated, single-subject study; 3 = comparison group but not clinical trial; 4 = no control group. Effect size: a = .81+, large; b = .51 to .80, medium; c = .21 to .50, small; d = .20 or less. CBT = cognitive behavior therapy; ADHD = attention-deficit/hyperactivity disorder; ODD = oppositional defiant disorder; CD = conduct disorder.
[a]Over 12 months. [b]See side effects and risk–benefit discussion.

also with infrequent weight gain. Divalproex sodium also has been found effective in ameliorating CD symptoms. Only one well-controlled study has been conducted to date (Steiner, Petersen, Saxena, Ford, & Matthews, 2003), although there are several small controlled and poorly controlled studies or case series attesting to some beneficial effect (see Steiner et al., 2003). For children with comorbid ADHD and ODD or CD, the combination of stimulant medication (e.g., methylphenidate) and clonidine is associated with improvements in symptoms of both disorders (e.g., Hazell & Stuart, 2003).

Minimal evidence is available for psychopharmacological treatment of ODD, except in cases in which comorbid ADHD is present. The Multimodal Treatment of ADHD (MTA) study indicated that children with ADHD and ODD responded best to medication treatment (i.e., psychostimulants) with or without the concomitant use of behavioral interventions (Jensen et al., 2001). Further, as previously mentioned, the combination of methylphenidate and clonidine may lead to reduction of both ADHD and ODD symptoms. One controlled study suggested that atomoxetine also may reduce symptoms of both disorders, especially at higher dosages (Newcorn, Spencer, Biederman, Milton, & Michelson, 2005).

Strength of Evidence

Pharmacological effects on aggression and conduct problems are in the small-to-moderate range, except for lithium effects on aggression, which are in the large range. Psychotropic medication (primarily lithium) may reduce aggression and stabilize mood in children and adolescents with CD. Stimulants and the combination of stimulants plus clonidine may address ODD symptoms in children with comorbid ADHD and ODD. In general, however, effect sizes for psychosocial interventions are larger than effect sizes for psychotropic medication with this population.

Side Effects

All of the medications used to treat aggression and conduct problems are associated with potential adverse side effects that, though rare, can be relatively serious. Side effects of lithium can include polyuria, polydipsia, motor tremor, increased appetite, dry mouth, general muscular weakness, and memory reduction (Henry, 2002; Luby & Singareddy, 2003). Risperidone, haloperidol, and other neuroleptic medications can be associated with serious extrapyramidal side effects (e.g., tardive dyskinesia) as well as headache, nausea, and drowsiness, not to mention the potentially lethal neuroleptic malignant syndrome (Edwards & Pople, 2002; Leucht, Pitschel-Walz, Abraham, & Kissling, 1999). Divalproex sodium can lead to a variety of side effects, including abdominal pain, headache, dizziness, drowsiness, and memory difficulties. Possible side effects of clonidine include sedation, lethargy, dry mouth, and low blood pressure (Connor, 2005a). Stimulants can be associated with a range of side effects, such as loss of appetite, sleep disturbance, headaches, stomachaches, and possibly motor tics (Connor, 2005b). Atomoxetine can lead to stomachaches, nausea, decreased appetite, and weight loss (Christman et al., 2004). As discussed in the previous chapter, the U.S. Food and Drug Administration (2005) issued a warning that atomoxetine may increase the risk of suicidal thinking in children and adolescents with ADHD; this risk is approximately 0.4%. Potential side effects associated with combined medication protocols have not been investigated extensively.

COMBINED INTERVENTIONS

Very few studies have specifically evaluated the effects of combined psychosocial and medication treatment protocols for children with ODD or CD. Kolko, Bukstein, and Barron (1999) examined the separate and incremental effects of two doses of methylphenidate and behavior modification in 16 children with ADHD and CD or ODD in the context of a partial hospitalization program. Although there were considerable individual differences in treatment response, both treatments were associated with positive effects in isolation and in combination. In similar fashion, the MTA study (Jensen et al., 2001) found that children with comorbid ADHD and ODD or CD showed positive behavioral response to carefully titrated stimulant medication with or without adjunctive psychosocial intervention. Alternatively, children with ADHD and multiple comorbid disorders (ODD, CD, or anxiety disorder) responded optimally to the combined medication and psychosocial treatment protocol (Jensen et al., 2001).

Strength of Evidence

The combination of psychosocial (behavioral) and pharmacological interventions for children with comorbid ADHD and ODD or CD leads to moderate-to-large effect size reductions for ADHD symptoms. Effect sizes for changes in aggression, oppositional behavior, and conduct problems are in the small-to-moderate range (MTA Cooperative Group, 1999a, 1999b).

Limitations

Given the lack of research on combined interventions for ODD/CD, minimal information is available regarding the specific limitations of combined treatment protocols. Side effects of medication and psychosocial treatments are presumed to be similar to those found for unimodal treatment but may be attenuated to the extent that lower dosages of each can be used when treatments are combined. It is probable that combined treatment is more costly, although detailed cost-effectiveness data comparing combined and unimodal treatment approaches are lacking.

DIVERSITY

Most treatment outcome studies for children and adolescents with ODD or CD have been conducted with White boys. Very few studies have examined differential treatment response across gender and ethnic groups. There is a higher prevalence of disruptive behavior disorders in boys; however, girls with CD may be at greater risk for comorbid internalizing symptoms (Keenan, Loeber, & Green, 1999). Further, although precursors of CD overlap with boys, some predictor variables may be specific to girls (e.g., emotionality, experience of empathy and guilt), and aggression may be manifested differently (i.e., through indirect or relational aggression rather than physical aggression; Kann & Hanna, 2000).

Although few studies have specifically examined gender differences in treatment response, investigators have speculated that interventions focused on peer relationships rather than gang involvement may be more effective for girls with CD (Kann & Hanna, 2000). Further, it is possible that family factors (e.g., parenting style) may predict parent training outcomes to a greater degree in girls than in boys (Webster-Stratton, 1996).

Differences in treatment outcome between ethnic and racial groups require further study, although preliminary research examining potential moderators of intervention outcome has not found differences between African American and White children (e.g., Lochman & Wells, 2004). Low socioeconomic status (SES), especially for single-parent families, is associated with lower response to parent training interventions (Reyno & McGrath, 2006). Lower rates of parental participation and treatment adherence in low-SES families may account for negative treatment outcomes. Further research examining treatment effects and outcomes by diversity variables is necessary.

RISK–BENEFIT ANALYSIS

No studies have formally analyzed benefits versus risks for pharmacological or psychosocial treatments for ODD or CD. Potentially significant side effects, though rare, can occur with psychopharmacological interventions. There are fewer risks associated with behavioral interventions, which include feasibility and resource concerns and possible social contagion effects of group-based treatments (Dishion & Dodge, 2005). The latter have only been found for young adolescents and on some dependent measures, and recent meta-analytic tests have not found overall support for iatrogenic or deviancy training effects in group interventions for children with ODD and CD (Weiss et al., 2005). Given the larger effect sizes associated with psychosocial interventions, these are preferred as first-line treatments over psychotropic medications.

FUTURE DIRECTIONS

There are several important directions for future investigations of treatments for children with ODD or CD. More clinical trials are necessary for the purpose of assisting practitioners in implementing interventions that are evidence-based as well as community-based. In addition, more studies need to examine treatment effects for children and adolescents from diverse backgrounds to identify specific risk factors, treatment predictors, treatment modalities, and outcomes associated with background factors (e.g., gender, race, SES, and ethnicity). Finally, given the complexity and intractability of disruptive behavior disorders, more investigations of combined treatments need to be conducted to elucidate effective combinations of psychosocial interventions, medications, or both across home, school, and community settings. These disorders often lead to long-term antisocial behavior at great cost to individuals and society. Efforts by child and pediatric psychologists would be well spent in this area, the savings probably measured on a per inmate–per year cost to society.

4

TOURETTE'S AND TIC DISORDERS

According to the *Diagnostic and Statistical Manual of Mental Disorders* (4th ed., text rev.; American Psychiatric Association, 2000), a diagnosis of *Tourette's disorder* (TD) requires the presence of multiple motor tics and at least one vocal tic, although not necessarily concurrently, for at least 12 months. Frequent motor or vocal tics, but not both, of at least 12 months duration warrant a diagnosis of *chronic motor* or *vocal tic disorder*. Collectively, these two disorders are referred to as *chronic tic disorder* (CTD). *Transient tic disorder*, characterized by mild tics present for at least 1 month but not more than 12 months, rarely requires pharmacological intervention and is not considered further in this review. In all cases, tic onset must be before age 18. Community prevalence estimates for TD in the United States range from 0.1% to 1%, rising to 1% to 2% when chronic motor or vocal tic disorder is also included (Scahill, Sukhodolsky, Williams, & Leckman, 2005). Coprolalia, often portrayed as the defining symptom of TD, is, in fact, relatively rare, occurring in fewer than 10% of individuals with this diagnosis (American Psychiatric Association, 2000).

The clinical course of TD is typically marked at onset by simple motor tics such as eye blinking and facial or head and neck tics beginning around age 6 or 7. This is followed by the development of vocal tics and a rostral-caudal progression of increasingly complex motor tics over several years. Tics usually follow a fluctuating course characterized by occasional bouts of increased tic frequency and severity interspersed with periods of relative quiescence. In most cases, CTD follows a fluctuating yet generally worsening course, reaching maximum severity in late childhood followed by a significant decrease in severity throughout adolescence and, in up to 50% of cases, complete remission by adulthood (Leckman et al., 1998). Comorbid attention-deficit/hyperactivity disorder, obsessive–compulsive disorder, anxiety, depression, and learning difficulties are common in youngsters with CTD and may account for much of the functional impairment seen in these cases (Freeman et al., 2000).

PSYCHOSOCIAL INTERVENTIONS

Numerous psychosocial approaches have been reported for the treatment of CTD, including contingency management, massed practice, relaxation training, hypnosis, self-monitoring, awareness training, exposure with response prevention (ERP), and habit reversal training (HRT; see reviews by A. A. Peterson, Campise, & Azrin, 1994; Piacentini & Chang, 2001). Although psychoeducation and social support are listed in the medical literature as the first-line psychosocial interventions (Leckman et al., 1999), HRT has received the most empirical attention and support (A. A. Peterson, 2007). HRT is a multicomponent intervention that first teaches individuals methods to increase awareness of their tics and urges to tic, and then instructs them on using a competing response (e.g., isometric tensing of muscles opposite to the tic movements) contingent on tic or urge expression (Azrin & Nunn, 1973). Treatments such as relaxation training and stress management, social support, and contingency management procedures, when paired with HRT, serve to address environmental and intrapersonal tic disorders and enhance compliance.

HRT demonstrated durable benefits for youngsters with CTD in a series of single-subject and multiple-baseline design studies and in a small controlled trial (Piacentini & Chang, 2006), but published between-groups design data from this age group are very limited. Only two of the six published randomized between-groups studies of HRT included children (Azrin & Peterson, 1990; Verdellen, Keijsers, Cath, & Hoogduin, 2004), and neither report provided sufficient detail to examine outcome by age. Of interest, Verdellen and associates found that ERP, most commonly used in the treatment of obsessive–compulsive disorder, is equally effective as HRT for tic reduction in their mixed-age study. Of the remaining psychosocial approaches, only contingency management procedures have generated enough empirical support to warrant consideration of use (A. L. Peterson, 2007). A randomized controlled, multisite trial (the Comprehensive Behavioral Intervention for Tics Study, or CBIT) funded by the National Institute of Mental Health

(NIMH) comparing a combined HRT plus contingency management approach to psychoeducation plus supportive therapy for childhood CTD should significantly enhance the psychosocial treatment evidence base for these disorders when completed in 2007. Table 4.1 provides a summary of treatment efficacy for CTD.

Strength of Evidence

Moderate effect sizes occurred for psychosocial treatment of chronic tic disorder most notably with HRT. These effects seem to be fairly durable, with continuing benefits demonstrated out to 1-year posttreatment. HRT also appears to be beneficial for tic-related functional impairment, as measured by the Yale Global Tic Severity Scale overall impairment scale (Leckman et al., 1999). However, this scale is relatively limited in scope. Less well documented than HRT, exposure (a procedure entailing having the child withhold tic behavior when the premonitory urge occurs) plus response prevention and contingency management approaches still seem to be moderately effective for the acute reduction of tic severity.

Limitations

Although a number of single-case, small-case series, and laboratory analogue studies document the benefits of behavior therapy for CTD, data from controlled psychosocial treatment trials that included children and adolescents are limited. Almost all of these studies contain mixed child and adult samples, and findings are rarely broken down by age. Clinical implementation and study of behavioral treatments have also been hampered by resistance to this form of treatment within the medical community and the lack of clinicians trained in these techniques. The psychosocial treatment literature contains insufficient information to ascertain the moderating effects of comorbidity and symptom severity on outcome, which is unfortunate given that these two factors often drive clinic referral. Although HRT can be associated with transient distress associated with increased tic awareness, more serious or long-term adverse effects have not been found for this treatment.

PHARMACOLOGICAL INTERVENTIONS

The relatively large number of different medications used to treat CTD over the years highlights the difficulty in achieving meaningful symptomatic relief in the absence of significant adverse side effects (Sandor, 2003). The most well-studied pharmacological agents for childhood CTD include the dopamine receptor blockers (typical neuroleptics): haloperidol and pimozide; the atypical neuroleptics: risperidone and ziprasidone; and the alpha$_2$-

TABLE 4.1
Treatment Efficacy for Chronic Tic Disorder, Including Tourette's Disorder

Treatment	Acute		Long term[a]		Side effects[b]
	Strength of evidence and effect size, Primary symptoms	Strength of evidence and effect size, Functional outcomes	Strength of evidence and effect size, Primary symptoms	Strength of evidence and effect size, Functional outcomes	
Psychosocial					
HRT	2a–c	2c	No data	No data	May be associated with transient tic increase.
ERP	3b	No data	No data	No data	Attempts to resist tic expression may lead to discomfort.
Contingency management	2c	No data	No data	No data	Potentially time consuming, questionable generalizability.
Medication					
Alpha$_2$ agonists					Sedation, dry mouth, headache, irritability, dysphoria, postural hypotension; guanfacine associated with less risk of sedation.
Clonidine	2c–d, Mild to moderate tics, ADHD	2c–d	No data	No data	
Guanfacine	2b–c, Tics, ADHD	2c–d	No data	No data	

Neuroleptics					Sedation, cognitive dulling, akathisia, EPS, ECG effects, risk of tardive dyskinesia, dysphoria; pimozide associated with less severe sedation and EPS.
Haloperidol	1b, Tics	No data	No data	No data	
Pimozide	1c, Tics	No data	No data	No data	
Atypical neuroleptics					Sedation, weight gain, EPS, galactorrhea, dysphoria, increased risk of hepatoxicity and diabetes mellitus; neuroleptic malignancy syndrome; ziprasidone less likely to cause weight gain than risperidone.
Risperidone	1b Tics	No data	No data	No data	
Ziprasidone	2b–c, Tics	No data	No data	No data	
Atomoxetine	2c, Tics, ADHD	No data	No data	No data	Stomachaches, nausea, decreased appetite, weight loss, risk of increased suicidal thinking.
Combination					
CBT + SSRI (sertraline)	No data	No data	No data	No data	No data

Note. Across all treatment studies for each type of child psychopathology, we used guidelines put forth by J. Cohen (1988): Strength of evidence: 1 = replicated clinical trial or large-body, single-subject study; 2 = controlled clinical trial or replicated, single-subject study; 3 = comparison group but not clinical trial; 4 = no control group. Effect size: a = .81+, large; b = .51 to .80, medium; c = .21 to .50, small; d = .20 or less. HRT = habit reversal training; ERP = exposure with response prevention; ADHD = attention-deficit/hyperactivity disorder; EPS = extrapyramidal symptoms; ECG = electrocardiograph; CBT = cognitive behavior therapy; SSRI = selective serotonin reuptake inhibitor.
[a] Over 12 months. [b] See side effects and risk–benefit discussion.

adrenergic agonists: clonidine and guanfacine (Cheng-Shannon, McGough, Pataki, & McCracken, 2004; Sandor, 2003; Zinner, 2004). Randomized controlled trials of between-groups or crossover designs have been published for each of these agents (Cummings, Singer, Krieger, Miller, & Mahone, 2002; Gaffney et al., 2002; Gilbert, Batterson, Sethuraman, & Sallee, 2004; Sallee et al., 2000; Sallee, Nesbitt, Jackson, Sine, & Sethuraman, 1997; Scahill et al., 2001; Shapiro et al., 1989; Singer et al., 1995; Tourette's Syndrome Study Group, 2002). Although characterized by relatively small sample sizes and brief duration, these studies suggest at least moderate treatment effects for the typical and atypical neuroleptics and guanfacine, with more equivocal support for clonidine. Several other agents, including atomoxetine, a selective noradrenergic reuptake inhibitor; mecamylamine, a nicotinergic receptor antagonist; and botulinum toxin are being used with some frequency for childhood CTD despite limited empirical support and concerns for safety (McCracken et al., 2003; Sandor, 2003; Zinner, 2004). The long-term efficacy and safety of psychopharmacological treatments for childhood CTD are underresearched.

Strength of Evidence

The strongest evidence for efficacy in tic suppression belongs to the dopamine-blocking agents: haloperidol and risperidone. Both of these agents has shown benefit in at least two controlled trials. Unfortunately, and as noted elsewhere, these agents are also associated with adverse event profiles serious enough to limit their utility as first-line interventions. Among the alpha$_2$-adrenergic agonists, the strength of evidence favors guanfacine over clonidine. Both clonidine and atomoxetine have demonstrated modest benefit in children and adolescents with comorbid tic disorder and ADHD. However, methodological limitations related to sample recruitment and attrition rates raise concerns regarding the generalizability of these findings (Gilbert, 2006). With the possible exception of ziprasidone, which showed efficacy in one controlled trial, evidence supporting the use of other treatments for tic suppression is extremely limited.

Side Effects

Neuroleptic use is associated with a range of serious side effects, including sedation, cognitive dulling, weight gain, extrapyramidal symptoms, electrocardiograph (i.e., ECG) findings, akathisia, depression, and anxiety (Cheng-Shannon et al., 2004; Sandor, 2003; Zinner, 2004). The atypical neuroleptics, risperidone and ziprasidone, are thought to be associated with reduced risk of extrapyramidal symptoms and tardive dyskinesia, but risperidone is associated with significant weight gain. Among the typical neuroleptics, Sallee et al. (1997) reported that haloperidol was associated with 3 times the rate of serious side effects as pimozide in youngsters with CTD even though the two treatments did not differ in efficacy. Although many of the controlled child CTD neuroleptic trials reported relatively low rates of serious side effects, it must be noted that these trials were generally of insufficient duration, typically no more than 8 weeks, not enough to evaluate safety fully. The adverse side effects of long-term treatment with neuroleptic drugs have been well documented (Werry & Aman, 1999), particularly in adults, and their therapeutic effects in children are of concern. Clonidine and guanfacine have significantly less harmful side effects than the neuroleptics with sedation, headache, irritability, and an increased risk of postural hypotension (Zinner, 2004).

COMBINED INTERVENTIONS

Combined interventions for childhood CTD have yet to be systematically studied.

DIVERSITY

The potential moderating effects of gender, race, and ethnicity on treatment outcomes have not been examined for childhood CTD. By far, most (85%–95%) study samples have been White males (probably related in some part to the gender distribution of the disorder in the community). Further research examining treatment effects and outcomes by diversity variables and other populations is necessary.

RISK–BENEFIT ANALYSIS

Treatment of tics in children and adolescents has evolved significantly over the past 2 decades. In most cases, the decision to treat a child's tics is not simply based on their presence but on the extent to which they are distressing or physically harmful to the child or interfere with academic, social, and family functioning. From a psychopharmacological perspective, the level of tic reduction must be balanced with the increased risk of side effects at higher medication doses. Whether these risks are present with low doses is uncertain. Administering low doses of medication typically precludes eradication of tics by medication alone, and a more achievable goal of 40% to 50% reduction in tic severity is favored (Scahill, Chappell, King, & Leckman, 2000). Even though clonidine and guanfacine are less consistently effective than the neuroleptics in reducing tic severity, these agents are typically considered first-line medication treatments for all but the most severe tics because of their increased safety and tolerability.

Renewed attention to psychosocial management strategies for tic control, most notably HRT and contingency management approaches, has the potential to enhance treatment options dramatically for affected youngsters. Although controlled data for childhood CTD are limited, those data that do exist support HRT as a viable treatment option either alone or in combination with medication for youngsters with mild to moderately severe tic disorder. At present, unfortunately, access to treatments for CTD is extremely limited because of an insufficient supply of clinicians, including behavioral psychologists and child psychiatrists. Results from the ongoing NIMH-funded multisite child CBIT study may serve, however, to spur dissemination of HRT throughout the CTD treatment community with the goal of ultimately establishing this treatment as a front-line intervention. It is hoped that this, in turn, will encourage clinicians to enter this area of need so children with this disorder will have better access to treatment.

FUTURE DIRECTIONS

Although controlled data from children and adolescents are now available for at least six different pharmacological agents and two psychosocial interventions, treatment options for youngsters with CTD remain less than ideal because of the lack of highly efficacious medications, concerns with the safety and tolerability of existing medications, and the lack of clinicians trained in the use of HRT and other promising behavioral interventions. The negative side effect profiles associated with the most commonly used anti-tic medications make it mandatory to develop and test a broad range of psychosocial interventions for childhood CTD. Studies examining combined medication and psychosocial treatment approaches, including the identification of treatment sequencing strategies, are also needed. Research documenting the longer term efficacy and safety of existing treatments remains to be conducted. Studies examining the effect of demographic status (e.g., age, gender, race), comorbid psychopathology, and cognitive functioning on outcome are also necessary. In addition, little is known about the effect of existing treatments on psychosocial functioning, both acutely and over the long term. Finally, translational studies aimed at elucidating the mechanisms by which behavioral and psychopharmacological treatments operate are needed to guide the refinement of existing treatments and increase the development of more effective interventions.

5

OBSESSIVE–COMPULSIVE DISORDER

Obsessive–compulsive disorder (OCD) is generally a chronic and impairing condition with a prevalence of .5% to 2% in children and adolescents (Rapoport et al., 2000). Relatively heterogeneous at diagnosis, the most common OCD symptoms in childhood include fears of harm or other negative outcomes; concerns with germs, contamination, and illness; and ritualized and excessive washing, cleaning, counting, checking, and arranging. The clinical picture and treatment planning are often complicated by the presence of comorbid psychiatric disorders, most commonly other anxiety disorders, depression, attention-deficit/hyperactivity disorder, and tic disorders, seen in up to 75% of youngsters with primary OCD (D. A. Geller et al., 2000). Up to 40% of youngsters with OCD meet diagnostic criteria for the disorder up to 15 years after initial identification, with another 20% evidencing subclinical disturbance at follow-up (Stewart et al., 2004).

PSYCHOSOCIAL INTERVENTIONS

The most well-studied cognitive behavior therapy (CBT) for OCD regardless of age is exposure with response prevention (ERP; Meyer, 1966). From a learning theory perspective, OCD is thought to be maintained by negative reinforcement wherein performance of the compulsion is reinforced by its ability to alleviate anxiety or distress triggered by an associated obsession. ERP disrupts the negative reinforcement cycle and allows for habituation of associated anxiety by systematically triggering the obsession through in vivo or imaginal exposure while simultaneously encouraging the child to refrain from ritualizing (Kozak & Foa, 1997). Although the contribution of cognitive distortions, including excessive fears of harm and exaggerated responsibility for negative outcomes, is less clear for OCD in children and adolescents than in adults, some form of cognitive intervention has become relatively standard in the treatment of childhood OCD. These techniques are typically aimed at teaching children to recognize and relabel their obsessive fears as OCD and more accurately evaluate the likelihood of feared consequences. CBT for childhood OCD also typically includes additional treatment components such as psychoeducation, structured parental involvement, and built-in reward systems to enhance motivation and compliance with exposure and foster greater generalization of gains (March & Mulle, 1998; Piacentini & Langley, 2004). In addition to a number of small positive open trials, three randomized controlled trials, two of which compared CBT to medication, have now been published and provide additional support for the efficacy of CBT for childhood OCD (Barrett, Healy-Farrell, & March, 2004; de Haan, Hoogduin, Buitelaar, & Keijsers, 1998; Pediatric OCD Treatment Study Team, 2004).

Barrett et al. (2004) found that individual CBT and CBT with groups that included a family intervention component were superior to a wait-list control condition. Both modules led to an approximate 60% decrease in OCD symptom severity compared with no change for wait-list youngsters. This study supported the efficacy of CBT for youngsters with OCD, but the findings are tempered by the lack of a primary outcome measure integrating both child- and parent-report information. Also, the wait-list condition was only 4 to 6 weeks in duration. Contrary to expectation, treatment-related gains were not observed on any family measures. Observed gains were largely maintained at a 6-month follow-up of the active treatment groups.

In addition, a fourth controlled trial found individual CBT supplemented with weekly family CBT superior to relaxation training plus psychoeducation (Piacentini, 2004). In the first direct comparison of CBT and medication, CBT proved statistically superior to clomipramine, a serotonin reuptake inhibitor, in terms of both rate of response to treatment (66.7% vs. 50%) and degree of symptom reduction (59.9% vs. 33.4%; de Haan et al., 1998). Although controlled data regarding the long-term efficacy of CBT for childhood OCD are limited (e.g., Barrett et al., 2004), reviews of published open trials with children and adolescents (Piacentini, March, & Franklin, 2006) and controlled research with adults (J. S. Abramowitz, 1997) suggest that such gains may be durable. In spite of widespread clinical use, the efficacy of psychodynamic, supportive, and family therapy as well as other non-CBT psychosocial approaches has yet to be demonstrated for OCD in individuals of any age (Jenike, 1990; March, Leonard, & Swedo, 1995). Table 5.1 provides a summary of treatment efficacy for OCD.

Strength of Evidence

Multiple controlled trials provided strong evidence for the efficacy of exposure-based CBT for treating OCD in children and adolescents, and one controlled trial supported the durability of benefits up to 6 months posttreatment (Barrett et al., 2004). However, as previously noted, sufficient controlled data are necessary before the positive effects of CBT on psychosocial functioning or the incremental efficacy of adding a systematic family intervention component to individual child treatment can be established.

Limitations

Despite a significant expansion in the evidence base supporting the use of CBT for childhood OCD, several limitations of this form of treatment remain. One is the fact that many youngsters show less than adequate response to CBT, and potential moderators of treatment response remain to be identified. Also, the effect of treatment on functional outcomes remains poorly understood and inadequately researched. Despite theoretical reasons to include family members in treatment, the incremental efficacy of structured family involvement in therapy has yet to be established. In addition, similar to many childhood disorders, treatment studies for childhood OCD are likely to include participants who may not otherwise have sought treatment, which may affect the generalizability of findings to other clinical samples.

PHARMACOLOGICAL INTERVENTIONS

Numerous clinical trials sponsored by pharmaceutical companies have demonstrated the efficacy of selective serotonin reuptake inhibitors (SSRIs) and the tricyclic antidepressant clomipramine for the treatment of childhood OCD (Leonard, Ale, Freeman, Garcia, & Nigg, 2005). Fluoxetine, fluvoxamine, sertraline, and clomipramine have received U.S. Food and Drug Administration (FDA) approval for use in children and adolescents with this disorder. However, overall medication efficacy is relatively modest, with active treatment typically yielding an average 30% to 40% decrease in OCD symptom severity (March & Curry, 1998). A recent meta-analysis of 12 published randomized placebo-controlled medication trials for childhood OCD (1,044 participants) showed an effect size of 0.46 with clomipramine, which was superior to the SSRIs (D. A. Geller et al., 2003).

TABLE 5.1
Treatment Efficacy for Obsessive–Compulsive Disorder

Treatment	Acute		Long term[a]		Side effects[b]
	Strength of evidence and effect size, Primary symptoms	Strength of evidence and effect size, Functional outcomes	Strength of evidence and effect size, Primary symptoms	Strength of evidence and effect size, Functional outcomes	
Psychosocial					
Exposure-based CBT Individual	1a, Obsessions, compulsions	1c, General functioning	4b, Continued efficacy to 18 months	No data	Exposure-triggered anxiety uncomfortable for some; intolerable in rare instances (mediator of efficacy).
Group	2a	2d	No data	No data	Exposure-triggered anxiety uncomfortable for some; intolerable in rare instances (mediator of efficacy).
Medication					
SSRIs and clomipramine	1b–c, Obsessions, compulsions	1b, General function	4b, Continued efficacy to 12 months of continued use	No data	Agitation, nausea, and suicidality (recent FDA warning). Sedation, fainting, seizures, tremor, weight gain for clomipramine.

Combination of CBT + SSRI (sertraline)	2a, Obsessions, compulsions	No data	No data	No data	Same as monotherapies.

Note. Across all treatment studies for each type of child psychopathology, we used guidelines put forth by J. Cohen (1988): Strength of evidence: 1 = replicated clinical trial or large-body, single-subject study; 2 = controlled clinical trial or replicated, single-subject study; 3 = comparison group but not clinical trial; 4 = no control group. Effect size: a = .81+, large; b = .51 to .80, medium; c = .21 to .50, small; d = .20 or less. CBT = cognitive behavior therapy; SSRI = selective serotonin reuptake inhibitor; FDA = U.S. Food and Drug Administration.
[a]Over 12 months. [b]See side effects and risk–benefit discussion.

Potential clomipramine-induced cardiotoxicity, however, contraindicates use of this medication as a first- or even second-line treatment (March, Frances, Carpenter, & Kahn, 1997). The SSRIs did not differ from each other in these studies (D. A. Geller et al., 2003). As mentioned previously, SSRIs also have their own adverse side effects. SSRIs reduce OCD-related functional impairment significantly, at least over the short term (D. A. Geller, Hoog, et al., 2001; Liebowitz et al., 2002).

Although a significant proportion of medication responders continue to meet criteria for clinically significant OCD following acute treatment, Cook et al. (2001) conducted a 1-year extension trial, the outcome of which suggested that treatment gains may continue to accrue over time. These findings are tempered by high rates of sample attrition and the fact that youngsters in the extension trial were allowed to participate in concomitant psychotherapy during this phase of the study. Symptom recurrence following medication discontinuation has not been systematically studied but is expected to be likely (Leonard et al., 2005).

Strength of Evidence

The efficacy of SSRIs for treating OCD in children and adolescents has been demonstrated in a number of large-scale controlled trials. On the basis of D. A. Geller et al.'s (2003) meta-analysis, however, the overall efficacy of pharmacotherapy for this disorder can be described only as modest.

Side Effects

As in clinical trials of anxiety without OCD, SSRIs tend to be relatively well tolerated in children and adolescents with OCD. The most commonly reported SSRI-related side effects include nausea, diarrhea, insomnia, loss of appetite, sedation, tremor, sexual dysfunction, and disinhibition (Leonard et al., 2005), but these are often transient in nature. In some blinded trials, SSRI-related attrition rates do not differ between the active and placebo treatment groups (March & Curry, 1998). As noted earlier in this book, however, FDA findings of an association between antidepressant use and increased risk of suicidality in children and adolescents have dramatically altered the parameters of medication use in this age group (U.S. Food and Drug Administration, 2005). The cardiotoxicity of clomipramine also necessitates maximum caution.

COMBINED INTERVENTIONS

The Pediatric OCD Treatment Study Team (2004) trial provided the only controlled data on the efficacy of combined (CBT plus medication) treatment for youngsters with OCD. This trial used a multicenter approach to compare CBT, sertraline, and their combination with pill placebo in 112 OCD youngsters ages 7 to 17 years. Using an intent-to-treat analytic strategy, all three active treatments significantly outperformed pill placebo. In addition, the combination of CBT and sertraline was found superior to CBT or sertraline, which did not differ from one another. However, a significant advantage was found for the two CBT conditions using "excellent response" as the outcome (combination 54%, CBT 39%, sertraline 21%, and placebo 3%). Study results were tempered by a significant site by treatment interaction in which CBT alone was equivalent to combination therapy at one site but not at the other. This suggests that, under certain circumstances, optimal CBT may preclude the need for any medication.

Strength of Evidence

Although the superiority of combined CBT plus medication to medication alone was clearly demonstrated by the Pediatric OCD Treatment Study Team (2004) trial, the potential superiority of combined treatment to CBT alone is much less clear. Effect sizes, calculated for each active treatment as compared to placebo, did not significantly differ between combined treatment (1.40) and CBT only (0.97) but were significantly different for combined treatment and medication only (0.67).

Limitations

The Pediatric OCD Treatment Study Team (2004) trial is the only controlled examination of combined treatment efficacy for childhood OCD to date. Moreover, this trial focused solely on acute efficacy, so information regarding the impact of combined treatment on functional outcomes or the durability of response, even over the short term, is not available. Finally, even though combined treatment in the trial was associated with a significant decrease in OCD severity, the 54% excellent response rate for this condition suggests that close to half of the individuals receiving combined treatment continued to experience some level of clinically meaningful OCD symptoms.

DIVERSITY

Gender and ethnicity have not been investigated as potential moderators of treatment response for either psychosocial or psychopharmacological interventions. Further research examining treatment effects and outcomes by diversity variables is warranted.

RISK–BENEFIT ANALYSIS

Although the efficacy of CBT and psychopharmacological approaches are well supported for adults with OCD (e.g., J. S. Abramowitz, 1997), sufficient data to evaluate the comparative efficacy and safety of psychosocial and psychopharmacological treatments for OCD in children and adolescents are only now becoming available (J. S. Abramowitz, Whiteside, & Deacon, 2005; D. A. Geller et al., 2003). On the basis of available efficacy and safety data, the risk–benefit balance clearly favors cognitive–behavioral intervention over medication for the treatment of child and adolescent OCD. This has led to the consensual clinical recommendation that CBT be implemented as the first-line treatment of choice, adding medication only if necessary, for OCD in children and adolescents (Pediatric OCD Treatment Study Team, 2004).

FUTURE DIRECTIONS

Despite the relatively robust effect sizes noted for CBT and combined treatment, a substantial proportion of children and adolescents in both the CBT and medication trials previously noted demonstrated a less than optimal response. Evidence-based intervention strategies need to be developed and tested for these youngsters as well as for those whose clinical picture is complicated by higher levels of OCD symptom severity or significant diagnostic comorbidity. More data on the ability of existing treatments to affect psychosocial functioning positively are also needed. In addition, controlled research is needed that examines the critical components of CBT for childhood OCD and the mechanisms of action for this treatment. For example, the efficacy of primarily cognitive interventions has garnered some support in the adult literature (e.g., J. S. Abramowitz, 1997), but this issue needs to be addressed in younger populations. Even though the impact of child OCD on family functioning is relatively well documented (e.g., Piacentini, Bergman, Keller, & McCracken, 2003; Waters & Barrett, 2000), family participation in child treatment has not yet been shown to enhance either child outcomes or family functioning (e.g., Barrett et al., 2004). Additional research is needed to establish the role of the family in child treatment (Barmish & Kendall, 2005).

6

ANXIETY DISORDERS

Anxiety disorders are among the most common mental health conditions affecting youths and include *generalized anxiety disorder* (GAD), *posttraumatic stress disorder* (PTSD), *separation anxiety disorder* (SAD), *selective mutism*, *specific phobia*, and *social anxiety disorder* (SoAD). Epidemiological studies estimate the prevalence of impairing anxiety disorders at greater than 10%, with four of five large surveys estimating prevalence to be 12% to 20% (Achenbach, Howell, McConaughy, & Stanger, 1995; Costello & Angold, 1995; Pine, 1994; Shaffer, Fisher, Dulcan, & Davies, 1996). Although anxiety has been historically considered fairly innocuous and developmentally normal, childhood anxiety disorders are associated with significant impairment and interfere with school performance, family functioning, and social functioning (Benjamin, Costello, & Warren, 1990). They can be as impairing in many ways as disruptive behavior disorders (Ialongo, Edelsohn, Werthamer-Larsson, Crockett, & Kellam, 1994). Moreover, anxiety in childhood predicts adult anxiety disorders, major depression, suicide attempts, and psychiatric hospitalization (Ferdinand & Verhulst, 1995; Pine, 1994). Retrospective and prospective studies confirm that anxiety disorders have an early onset and a chronic and fluctuating course through adolescence and into adulthood (Costello, Mustillo, Erkanli, Keeler, & Angold, 2003; Eaton, 1995; Kessler et al., 1994).

Investigators conducting controlled psychosocial and medication trials for childhood anxiety disorder have focused on GAD, SAD, and SoAD collectively because these three disorders share a common underlying construct of anxiety; are highly comorbid with each other, both cross-sectionally and over time; infrequently occur as isolated conditions; and show similar familial relationships with adult anxiety and depressive disorders (Gurley, Cohen, Pine, & Brook, 1996; P. C. Kendall & Brady, 1995; Last, Hersen, Kazdin, Orvaschel, & Perrin, 1991). Cognitive behavior therapy (CBT) and pharmacological interventions with selective serotonin reuptake inhibitors (SSRIs) are effective for treating children and adolescents with these three disorders. As such, the level of support for these treatments can be considered good to excellent.

PSYCHOSOCIAL INTERVENTIONS

Several randomized controlled clinical trials found CBT superior to wait-list control for relieving primary anxiety symptoms associated with GAD, SAD, and SoAD even to the point that a large percentage of treated youngsters were indistinguishable from peers who did not have these disorders (Barrett, Dadds, & Rapee, 1996; P. C. Kendall, 1994; P. C. Kendall et al., 1997; P. C. Kendall & Southam-Gerow, 1996; Last, Hansen, & Franco, 1998). CBT was also superior to wait-list in enhancing social competence in children and adolescents with SoAD.

In their systematic review of the CBT literature, Cartwright-Hatton, Roberts, Chitsabesan, Fothergill, and Harrington (2004) identified 10 published trials (total of 608 youngsters) comparing individual CBT with an inactive control condition for childhood anxiety disorder (excluding trials focusing solely on simple phobia, PTSD, and obsessive–compulsive disorder [OCD]). Using remission of the primary anxiety diagnosis as the outcome of interest, these investigators found pooled remission rates of 56.5% for CBT and 34.8% for wait-list, which yielded a pooled odds ratio of 3.3 (95% confidence interval = 1.9–5.6) in favor of CBT. The long-term durability of positive treatment effects is less well known. Although positive gains have been reported up to 7 years posttreatment (Barrett, Duffy, Dadds, & Rapee, 2001; P. C. Kendall, Safford, Flannery-Schroeder, & Webb, 2004), these data were obtained through single-source telephone interviews, in an uncontrolled fashion, and covered a relatively narrow set of outcome variables.

Similar to childhood OCD, the role of parental involvement in the treatment of childhood anxiety requires additional research (Barmish & Kendall, 2005; Silverman & Berman, 2001). Although a number of controlled trials have reported the benefits of family involvement in CBT for childhood anxiety versus individual treatment only, findings have not been consistent within or across the different studies (Barrett et al., 1996; Cobham,

Dadds, & Spence, 1998; Nauta, Scholing, Emmelkamp, & Minderaa, 2003; Spence, Donovan, & Brechman-Toussaint, 2000; J. J. Wood, Piacentini, Southam-Gerow, Chu, & Sigman, 2006). Moreover, the few longitudinal data available cast doubt on the durability of this benefit (Barrett et al., 2001). In terms of group treatment, Silverman, Kurtines, Ginsburg, Weems, Lumpkin, and Carmichael (1999) demonstrated the efficacy of CBT administered in group format (GCBT) for youngsters with social anxiety, overanxious, or generalized anxiety disorders. Sixty-four percent of children receiving GCBT were able to reduce their primary anxiety disorder symptoms compared with only 13% in the wait-list condition. On a similar note, Beidel, Turner, and Morris (2000) found a group behavioral intervention based on skill enhancement helpful for children with SoAD.

The benefits of behavioral treatments (including systematic desensitization, reinforced practice, and participant modeling) in reducing the subjective fear and avoidance associated with specific phobias were reviewed by Davis and Ollendick (2005). Ost, Svensson, Hellstrom, and Lindwall (2001) found an intensive single-session CBT intervention to be more effective for specific phobia in children than a wait-list condition. In one of the few child CBT trials with an active comparison condition, Silverman, Kurtines, Ginsburg, Weems, Rabian, and Serafini (1999) found exposure-based contingency management (a behavioral intervention), exposure-based self-control (a CBT intervention), and psychoeducational-supportive therapy were equally efficacious for reducing specific phobia in a sample of 81 youngsters ages 6 to 16 years. The only other CBT trial with psychoeducation and supportive therapy also found psychoeducational-supportive therapy and CBT equally effective, in this case for reducing school refusal behavior (Last et al., 1998). For children with PTSD, CBT interventions are efficacious compared with wait-list or other non-CBT psychotherapeutic support (J. A. Cohen, Deblinger, Mannarino, & Steer, 2004; N. J. King et al., 2000; Stein et al., 2003). Table 6.1 provides a summary of treatment efficacy for anxiety disorders.

Strength of Evidence

Many investigators conducting controlled trials have documented the efficacy and durability of CBT and other behavior therapies for childhood anxiety disorders, whether delivered in individual, group, or family-based format, with effect sizes in the moderate-to-large range.

Limitations

Although the research strongly supports the efficacy of CBT for childhood anxiety disorders, certain limitations must be considered, especially

TABLE 6.1
Treatment Efficacy for Anxiety Disorders

Treatment	Acute		Long term[a]		
	Strength of evidence and effect size, Primary symptoms	Strength of evidence and effect size, Functional outcomes	Strength of evidence and effect size, Primary symptoms	Strength of evidence and effect size, Functional outcomes	Side effects[b]
Psychosocial					
Individual CBT	1a, Anxiety and avoidance symptoms	1a, Overall functioning	4a, Anxiety and avoidance symptoms	4a, Overall functioning, reduced risk of later substance use	Well tolerated but limited systematic data.
Individual + parent CBT	1a, Anxiety and avoidance symptoms	1a, Overall functioning	4a, Inconsistent findings regarding durability of benefit compared with individual CBT	4a, Overall functioning	
Medication					
SSRIs	1a–c, Anxiety and avoidance symptoms	1a–c, Social functioning	No data	No data	Can cause restlessness and gastrointestinal symptoms, associated with increased risk of suicidal behavior, black-box warnings.
Combination	No data	No data	No data	No data	

Note. Across all treatment studies for each type of child psychopathology, we used guidelines put forth by J. Cohen (1988): Strength of evidence: 1 = replicated clinical trial or large-body, single-subject study; 2 = controlled clinical trial or replicated, single-subject study; 3 = comparison group but not clinical trial; 4 = no control group. Effect size: a = .81+, large; b = .51 to .80, medium; c = .21 to .50, small; d = .20 or less. CBT = cognitive behavior therapy; SSRI = selective serotonin reuptake inhibitor.
[a]Over 12 months. [b]See side effects and risk–benefit discussion.

when comparing CBT with psychopharmacological trials (Compton, Burns, Egger, & Robertson, 2002). First, most CBT trials used wait-list (i.e., no treatment) control conditions, which provide no protection against the confound of therapist attention or positive expectations about treatment. In fact, as previously noted, the only two CBT trials with an active comparison treatment (i.e., psychoeducation and support) found the comparison treatment to perform as well as CBT. Although psychoeducation is an active component of CBT for anxiety, this raises questions regarding the specificity of CBT effects. Second, CBT research for child anxiety has typically limited data analysis to those participants who actually completed treatment (completer analysis) rather than the much more stringent practice of including all randomized individuals regardless of outcome (intent-to-treat analysis). Completer analyses are likely to overstate the actual efficacy of a given treatment because they fail to account for individuals who dropped out of treatment because of perceived lack of efficacy, dislike of the treatment or therapist, adverse treatment effects, or other reasons.

PHARMACOLOGICAL INTERVENTIONS

Although a number of pharmacological agents have been evaluated for childhood anxiety disorders, efficacy data strongly favor SSRIs, at least for the treatment of GAD, SAD, and SoAD. Imipramine, one of the first medications tested for childhood anxiety, was superior to placebo for children with school avoidance (Gittelman-Klein & Klein, 1973), though not in children with SAD (Klein, Koplewicz, & Kanner, 1992). Because of its tolerability profile, risk of cardiotoxicity in overdose, and the availability of better tolerated medications (see Werry & Aman, 1999, for review), the use of imipramine has become rare.

Two small controlled trials failed to support the use of two benzodiazapines, clonazepam (Graae, Milner, Rizzotto, & Klein, 1994) and alprazolam (Simeon, Dinicola, Ferguson, & Copping, 1990). In contrast, a recent multisite placebo-controlled trial funded by the National Institute of Mental Health (NIMH) found fluvoxamine (an SSRI) highly efficacious and well tolerated in youngsters (ages 6–17 years) with GAD, SAD, and SoAD (Research Units on Pediatric Psychopharmacology [RUPP] Anxiety Study Group, 2001a, 2001b). Subsequent moderator analyses found that lower parent-reported child depression scores at baseline were associated with a more marked advantage of fluvoxamine over placebo. Youngsters with social phobia and greater overall illness severity at baseline were significantly less likely to improve regardless of treatment condition (RUPP Anxiety Study Group, 2003). Furthermore, Wagner, Berard, et al. (2004) found paroxetine (an SSRI) in children and adolescents with social phobia effective in a multisite controlled investigation. However, this medication is not currently recommended for use by children or adolescents because of safety concerns (GlaxoSmithKline, n.d.).

Smaller placebo-controlled trials support the efficacy of SSRIs fluoxetine and sertraline in children with GAD (Birmaher et al., 2003; Rynn, Siqueland, & Rickels, 2001). Data for medication efficacy for PTSD or specific phobia do not exist. However, Black and Uhde (1994) reported mixed findings from a small controlled trial of fluoxetine for selective mutism, a developmental variant of SoAD affecting mostly children under the age of 8 (Bergman & Piacentini, 2005). Few data are available on functioning or the durability of medication effects. Only limited data exist regarding the long-term use of SSRIs for childhood anxiety disorder, although 94% of acute phase positive responders to fluvoxamine retained their positive response without any dose changes over a 6-month follow-up period (RUPP Anxiety Study Group, 2002).

Strength of Evidence

Taken in combination, the relative lack of efficacy and adverse safety profiles of benzodiazapines and tricyclic antidepressants do not support their use in the treatment of children and adolescents with an anxiety disorder. In contrast, data from four controlled SSRI trials documented moderate to large positive effects for the acute reduction of the primary symptoms of SoAD, SAD, and GAD.

Side Effects

SSRIs tend to be relatively well tolerated in children and adolescents with anxiety. The most commonly reported SSRI-related side effects include nausea, diarrhea, insomnia, loss of appetite, sedation, tremor, sexual dysfunction, and disinhibition (Leonard, Ale, Freeman, Garcia, & Nigg, 2005). However, these effects are often transient in nature, and in some blinded trials, SSRI-related attrition rates do not differ between the active and placebo treatment groups (March & Curry, 1998). FDA findings of an association between antidepressant use and increased risk of suicidality in children and adolescents immediately changed applications of these medications for children.

COMBINED INTERVENTIONS

Little information is available on the relative efficacy of combined CBT and pharmacotherapy versus monotherapy for childhood anxiety. Bernstein et al. (2000) compared CBT monotherapy with the combination of CBT and imipramine for children with school refusal and comorbid depression and found the combination to be superior. A large NIMH-funded multisite trial, the Child/Adolescent Anxiety Multimodal Treatment Study (CAMS), is in progress to compare directly the effects of CBT, sertraline, and their combination in children and adolescents with GAD, SAD, and SoAD.

Strength of Evidence

Given that all subjects in the Bernstein et al. (2000) study also suffered from comorbid depression, this study does not directly address the benefits of combined treatment for the majority of children and adolescents with anxiety disorder. Generalizable evidence in this regard will have to wait for completion of the NIMH CAMS trial.

Limitations

The utility of the Bernstein et al. (2000) study is further limited by the fact that imipramine is associated with a host of adverse effects, including cardiac arrhythmia, and has even resulted in death (see Brown & Daly, in press). In addition, the efficacy of imipramine is equivocal at best with regard to management of anxiety disorders in children. These safety issues of imipramine mandate finding other treatment avenues.

DIVERSITY

As with most childhood disorders, the moderating effects of age, gender, and ethnicity on treatment outcome for anxiety disorders have been poorly studied. In many cases, insufficient sample size, wide age ranges, and the relatively homogeneous makeup of many study samples have hampered research on this topic. Barrett et al. (1996) reported a higher response rate for younger boys and girls whose parents also completed a 12-session family management program, compared with children whose parents did not receive treatment. However, as noted by Silverman and Berman (2001), this finding could be explained by the possible confounding of age with diagnosis (i.e., younger children are more likely to have SAD, which involves higher levels of parental involvement, and older children are more likely to have comorbid depressive symptoms).

For ethnicity, Hispanic or Latino youths have evidenced similar response rates to CBT as European American youths (Pina, Silverman, Fuentes, Kurtines, & Weems, 2003). The multisite RUPP fluvoxamine trial did not find child age, gender, race, ethnicity, parental education, or family income to moderate treatment outcome (RUPP Anxiety Study Group, 2003). Further research examining treatment effects and outcomes by diversity variables is necessary.

RISK–BENEFIT ANALYSIS

The primary risk–benefit consideration for childhood anxiety relates to the decision of whether or not to treat. Although often considered normative or of limited clinical significance, childhood anxiety disorders can be associated with considerable distress and impairment and lead to heightened risk for multiple adverse outcomes, including mood disturbance, substance abuse/dependence, suicidality, and poorer adult role performance (Ferdinand & Verhulst, 1995; Pine, 1994). Substantial evidence provides strong support for the efficacy of CBT in reducing the symptoms of childhood anxiety. In addition, data supporting the use of SSRI medication in anxious youngsters have recently emerged from two larger multisite and two smaller single-site trials. The efficacy of combined treatments (CBT plus medication) has yet to be published, but the research is under way. Unfortunately, studies directly comparing CBT and medication for childhood anxiety disorders without OCD do not yet exist.

Comparison of findings from the CBT and psychopharmacological literature is complicated by numerous design differences. These include the use of different treatment outcome measures (typically, remission of primary anxiety disorder symptoms in the CBT trials vs. better scores on the Clinical Global Impressions-Improvement Scale [Guy, 1976], a single-item clinician rating, in the medication studies) and the less common use of active comparison conditions and intent-to-treat analytic strategies by CBT researchers (Compton et al., 2004). Despite these differences, however, consensus strongly favors CBT alone as the first-line treatment of choice because of its larger database, greater durability of benefit associated with this treatment, and concerns about medication safety. Treatment with SSRI medication does remain a viable choice for youngsters who are unable to engage in or are nonresponsive to CBT or those for whom CBT is not readily available. The shortage of child psychiatrists in the United States may also mean medication treatment may be difficult to access as well.

FUTURE DIRECTIONS

Data from the ongoing NIMH CAMS trial should provide much-needed information about the comparative efficacy of CBT, SSRI medication, and their combination and guide treatment toward what works best for which youngsters under which circumstances. Additional studies are needed for better understanding of the optimal role of parents and other family members in treatment and to identify potential moderators of treatment response. The two CBT trials using psychoeducation as part of active comparison conditions found surprisingly high response rates to this intervention (Last et al., 1998; Silverman, Kurtines, Ginsburg, Weems, Rabian, & Serafini, 1999).

Expanded efforts are also needed to identify the mechanisms of action and critical components of CBT. Participants in child anxiety research trials, which typically take place in university settings, have been more likely to come from low-income and single-parent families and to have higher rates of externalizing diagnoses and other co-occurring psychiatric diagnoses than anxious youngsters treated in community settings (e.g., mental health centers, private practice; Southam-Gerow, Weisz, & Kendall, 2003). Children and adolescents with different but potentially complicating factors (e.g., low IQ, substance use, medical illness) also are typically excluded from clinical trials. Research needs to be conducted in these areas as well so that evidence-based treatments are available for youths with complicated presentations.

7

DEPRESSIVE DISORDERS AND SUICIDALITY

Clinical depression, defined to include *major depressive disorder* and *dysthymic disorder*, has been identified in children of all ages. Its prevalence rises sharply during adolescence, particularly among girls (e.g., Kessler, Avenevoli, & Merikangas, 2001; Petersen et al., 1993). By age 18, lifetime prevalence rates are approximately 20%, with significantly higher rates among girls (Hankin et al., 1998; Lewinsohn, Hops, Roberts, Seeley, & Andrews, 1993).

Depressive disorders are associated with substantial social and academic impairment (e.g., Puig-Antich et al., 1993), a wide range of comorbid psychopathology (Kovacs, 1996), increased risk for substance abuse (e.g., Kovacs, Goldston, & Gatsonis, 1993), and increased risk of attempted and completed suicide (Marttunen, Aro, Henriksson, & Lonnqvist, 1991; Rao, Weissman, Martin, & Hammond, 1993; Shaffer, Garland, Gould, Fisher, & Trautman, 1988). These disorders are often persistent, with a high risk of recurrence (DuBois, Felner, Bartels, & Silverman, 1995; Fleming, Boyle, & Offord, 1993; Kovacs, Obrosky, Gatsonis, & Richards, 1997; Lewinsohn, Clarke, Seeley, & Rohde, 1994).

Often associated with depressive disorders, suicidal thoughts and behaviors are reported by a substantial number of youths. In an administration of the Youth Risk Behavior Survey to a nationally representative sample, 8.5% of the total sample of high school students self-reported having attempted suicide in the past year (many of these were characterized by a low level of lethality), and 16.9% of the total sample reported having seriously considered making such an attempt (Grunbaum et al., 2004). Although suicidality is not limited to youths with depressive disorders, most adolescents with depressive disorders report significant suicidal ideation, and a significant minority report having made a suicide attempt during the course of their depression (Myers, McCauley, Calderon, & Treder, 1991).

This chapter excludes psychotic depression because of its relative rarity and the fact that children and adolescents with psychosis are routinely excluded from controlled intervention studies focusing on depression.

PSYCHOSOCIAL INTERVENTIONS

Interpersonal psychotherapy for adolescents (IPT-A) and cognitive behavior therapy (CBT) are the only psychosocial interventions for depression in children and adolescents that have been systematically examined. Although psychoeducation is not considered a primary treatment for depression, investigators have also begun to examine it as a psychosocial intervention for youths with depressive disorders and for their families.

Interpersonal Psychotherapy for Adolescents

IPT-A is a modification of the interpersonal psychotherapy originally developed for adult outpatients with depression by Klerman, Weissman, Rounsaville, and Chevron (1984). It addresses interpersonal issues common during adolescence, such as separation from parents, role transitions, authority conflicts, peer pressure and development of healthy peer relationships, death of a relative or friend, and the challenges associated with single-parent or stepparent families (Mufson, Moreau, Weissman, & Klerman, 1993). Using a focused, time-limited approach, the IPT therapist helps the adolescent understand and resolve the identified interpersonal issue. Although IPT-A has been modified for group settings (Mufson, Gallagher, Dorta, & Young, 2004), most published trials examined individual therapy.

Following a promising open clinical trial (Mufson et al., 1994) and 1-year follow-up study (Mufson & Fairbanks, 1996), Mufson, Weissman, Moreau, and Garfinkel (1999) conducted a randomized controlled 12-week clinical trial comparing IPT-A with clinical monitoring in a sample of 48 clinic-referred adolescents with major depression. Adolescents who received IPT-A reported a greater reduction in depressive symptoms and greater improvement in social functioning and problem-solving skills posttreatment. Adolescents who received IPT-A met the recovery criterion by 75%, compared with 46% of adolescents in the control condition. Despite study limitations, which include substantial attrition from the control condition and a marked difference between IPT-A and control conditions in therapist contact time, findings indicated that IPT-A was beneficial. In another published IPT-A effectiveness study, adolescents who met inclusion criteria for depression symptom severity (primarily Latina girls) were randomly assigned to receive either IPT-A or treatment-as-usual from school-based health clinicians (Mufson, Gallagher, et al., 2004). Adolescents treated with IPT-A showed greater symptom reduction and improvement in overall social functioning. Thus Mufson et al. have demonstrated the efficacy of IPT-A in two randomized controlled clinical trials.

Cognitive Behavior Therapy

Incorporating a variety of techniques, CBT for depression is a present-focused, time-limited, collaborative approach. It emphasizes the importance of a careful understanding or functional analysis of cognitive and behavioral factors related to initial symptoms. The CBT therapist generally aims to accomplish one or more of the following: reduce negatively distorted cognitions, improve problem-solving and coping skills, and increase the youth's involvement in healthy, pleasurable activities (e.g., Lewinsohn, Clarke, Hops, & Andrews, 1990). As described in Compton et al. (2004), CBT treatments often consist of required skill-building sessions and optional modular sessions for specific problems. Treatment may also involve parent and family sessions (e.g., Clarke, Rohde, Lewinsohn, Hops, & Seeley, 1999; Lewinsohn et al., 1990). Studies have incorporated variants of CBT, with some placing a greater emphasis on cognitive restructuring (Brent et al., 1997) and others taking a more behavioral and modular skills training approach, such as the Adolescent Coping With Depression Course (Lewinsohn & Clarke, 1984; Rohde, Lewinsohn, & Clarke, 2005).

Randomized controlled clinical trials comparing CBT with either no treatment or relaxation training have generally found CBT to be superior, irrespective of whether the studies provided CBT individually (A. Wood, Harrington, & Moore, 1996) or in groups (Clarke et al., 1999; Kahn, Kehle, Jenson, & Clark, 1990; Lewinsohn et al., 1990; Reynolds & Coats, 1986; Stark, Reynolds, & Kaslow, 1987; Weisz, Thurber, Sweeney, Proffitt, & LeGagnoux, 1997). One exception is a randomized controlled clinical trial that examined the relative efficacy of social competence training, an attention placebo control, and a no-treatment control for preadolescent children with depressive disorders (Liddle & Spence, 1990). There were no differences found among the groups, although the small sample of 31 children suggests severely limited statistical power, making it difficult to interpret these nonsignificant findings.

Other randomized controlled clinical trials, most of which have been conducted more recently, have compared CBT with active control conditions or treatments assumed to be active treatments for depression. These treatments include systemic family therapy or nondirective supportive therapy (Brent et al., 1997; Fine, Forth, Gilbert, & Haley, 1991), IPT (Rossello & Bernal, 1999), a life skills and tutoring intervention (Rohde, Clarke, Mace, Jorgensen, & Seeley, 2004), and selective serotonin reuptake inhibitors (SSRIs) in the Treatment for Adolescent Depression Study (TADS; 2004).

The TADS, described in greater detail in the section on combined interventions, was a large-scale multisite investigation that sampled adolescents with moderate to severe depression. Twelve-week clinical outcomes for the CBT arm were found not to differ from those of the pill placebo arm. In contrast to these findings, Brent et al. (1997) found better initial recovery rates for CBT than for systemic family therapy and supportive therapy, although treatment groups did not significantly differ in terms of remission, recovery, relapse, or recurrence across a 24-month follow-up period (Birmaher et al., 2000). Fine et al. (1991) found supportive therapy superior to behaviorally oriented CBT immediately posttreatment, with no differences evident at 9-month follow-up. Rossello and Bernal (1999) reported no differences in primary outcomes between CBT and IPT-A treatment groups, and Vostanis, Feehan, Grattan, and Bickerton (1996) found no difference between CBT and a nonfocused intervention. Even bibliotherapy (Ackerson, Scogin, McKendree-Smith, & Lyman, 1998) has shown promise as an intervention for adolescent depression but requires further study.

Although relatively small sample sizes make it difficult to draw firm conclusions, overall these investigators suggest that children and adolescents with depressive disorders respond similarly to different active psychosocial interventions. In fact, a recent comprehensive meta-analysis of psychotherapy for youths with depression showed small (mean effect size of .34) overall effects of weak durability (Weisz, McCarty, & Valeri, 2006). In this meta-analysis, cognitive approaches were neither better nor worse than noncognitive approaches. Note that results from meta-analyses may be limited by interpretation because the results may vary in accordance with the decisions of which data to analyze.

Psychoeducation

There is an absence of randomized controlled clinical trials examining the efficacy of psychoeducation as a stand-alone intervention for the families of children with depressive disorders, but it has been used as an adjunct to pharmacological interventions and as a component of many psychotherapeutic interventions for children and adolescents (e.g., Brent, Poling, McKain, & Baugher, 1993; Fristad, Gavazzi, Centolella, & Soldano, 1996; Geist, Heinmaa, Stephens, Davis, & Katzman, 2000; Goldberg-Arnold, Fristad, &

Gavazzi, 1999; C. A. King et al., 2006; Rotheram-Borus et al., 1996). In a study that provided a 2-hour psychoeducation session to the parents of 34 adolescents with depression, Brent, Kolko, Birmaher, Baugher, and Bridge (1999) found that psychoeducation was feasible, was positively received by families, and resulted in significant improvements in knowledge. Such psychoeducation has the potential to improve treatment adherence and outcome, particularly given the beneficial effects that have been demonstrated in studies of adult patients with affective disorders (e.g., C. M. Anderson et al., 1986). Although additional empirical studies are needed, it would seem ethically responsible to educate young patients and their parents on depression and its possible impact on functioning; alternative evidence-based treatments available; the potential risks, benefits, and discontinuation effects of specific recommended treatments; and the importance of close professional monitoring of physical status and safety.

Suicidal Ideation and Behavior

Despite the relatively high prevalence of suicidal behavior among youths, particularly adolescents, and the upsurge in national attention focused on the tragedy of youth suicide (e.g., *The Surgeon General's Call to Action to Prevent Suicide*; U.S. Public Health Service, 1999), the availability of evidence-based treatments for suicidal youths is extremely limited. Multisystemic therapy (MST; Henggeler, Schoenwald, Rowland, & Cunningham, 2002) is one of the few psychosocial interventions for suicidal youths to be evaluated in a randomized controlled clinical trial. MST is an intensive and time-limited home-based approach that centers on the family. In a study of 156 youths approved for psychiatric hospitalization due to suicidality, psychosis, or other threat of harm to self or others, Huey et al. (2004) found that MST was more effective than emergency hospitalization in decreasing youth-reported (but not parent-reported) suicide attempts. These data are promising despite the fact that the nonequivalency of MST and comparison groups at baseline (31% vs. 19% with histories of suicide attempts, respectively) makes the interpretation of differences in suicide attempts at posttreatment (14% vs. 9%) and 1-year follow-up (4% for both groups) somewhat difficult. MST was not effective in reducing suicidal ideation, hopelessness, or depression severity.

Other researchers conducting randomized controlled clinical trials with suicidal youths have shown either no significant effect for the experimental treatment or significant positive effects for only a subset of adolescents. In their comparison of group therapy (integration of CBT, dialectical behavior therapy [DBT], and psychodynamic approaches) with routine care, A. Wood, Trainor, Rothwell, Moore, and Harrington (2001) found that adolescents in group therapy were less likely to engage in repeated deliberate self-harm (two or more further incidents) up to the 7-month follow-up. In a study of a home-based family intervention for youths who had poisoned themselves, Harrington et al. (1998) found no difference between routine care and intervention groups at follow-up. Post hoc analyses, however, indicated that the intervention was linked to reduced suicidal ideation in youths without major depression.

Cotgrove, Zirinsky, Black, and Weston (1995) investigated the effect of giving suicidal youths a card permitting rehospitalization if needed and requested. They reported a nonsignificant reduction in suicide attempts for the experimental group at 1-year follow-up. C. A. King et al. (2006) are studying the efficacy of a social network intervention, the Youth-Nominated Support Team Intervention (YST), for suicidal adolescents who have been psychiatrically hospitalized because of acute suicidality. Although their large-scale preliminary study was primarily a feasibility trial, C. A. King et al. suggested possible YST-associated improvements in functioning for suicidal adolescent girls. A more rigorous randomized controlled clinical trial, incorporating an extensive risk management protocol, is ongoing to examine the efficacy of a modified version of the intervention.

Both DBT (Linehan, Armstrong, Suarez, Allmon, & Heard, 1991; Linehan, Heard, & Armstrong, 1993) and cognitive therapy (G. K. Brown et al., 2005) have shown effectiveness in reducing suicidal behavior in adults. Although randomized controlled clinical trials have not yet been conducted for DBT with adolescents, this strategy has shown some promise in preliminary trials with suicidal adolescents (Katz, Cox, Gunasekara, & Miller, 2004). On a similar note, a quasi-experimental study (Rotheram-Borus, Piacentini, Cantwell, Belin, & Song, 2000) found that an emergency room intervention for adolescent girls attempting suicide was associated with improved treatment adherence. Table 7.1 provides a summary of treatment efficacy for depressive disorders and suicidality for children and adolescents.

Strength of Evidence

The specific advantage of one psychosocial intervention over another in randomized controlled intervention trials has usually been small to none. The specific advantages of psychosocial interventions over wait list are generally moderate. The specific efficacy advantage of a psychosocial intervention (e.g., TADS) over placebo was nonexistent, but the harm of not treating was substantial. Although some psychosocial interventions for suicidal behavior are promising (e.g., MST), there have been methodological challenges and limitations in these intervention studies, so replication of the initial findings will be crucial. Studies documenting adverse effects associated with CBT were not found.

Limitations

Psychosocial interventions may not appeal to everyone because they involve the child or adolescent and often the parent(s), in collaborative work

TABLE 7.1
Treatment Efficacy for Depressive Disorders and Suicidality

	Acute		Long term[a]		
Treatment	Strength of evidence and effect size, Primary symptoms	Strength of evidence and effect size, Functional outcomes	Strength of evidence and effect size, Primary symptoms	Strength of evidence and effect size, Functional outcomes	Side effects[b]
Psychosocial					
IPT-A	1c, Depressive symptoms	1c, Social functioning	No data	No data	No data
CBT	1c, Depressive symptoms, suicidal ideation	No data	1–2c, Depressive symptoms	No data	No data
MST	2c–d, Suicide attempts	No data	No data	No data	No data
Medication					
Fluoxetine	1c, Depressive symptoms	1d	No data	No data	Agitation, irritability, insomnia, sedation, gastrointestinal problems, suicidality.
Other SSRIs	1d	1d	No data	No data	
Combination					
Fluoxetine + CBT	2a for depressive symptoms, 2c for suicidal ideation	No data	No data	No data	Insomnia, fatigue, gastrointestinal problems.

Note. Across all treatment studies for each type of child psychopathology, we used guidelines put forth by J. Cohen (1988): Strength of evidence: 1 = replicated clinical trial or large-body, single-subject study; 2 = controlled clinical trial or replicated, single-subject study; 3 = comparison group but not clinical trial; 4 = no control group. Effect size: a = .81+, large; b = .51 to .80, medium; c = .21 to .50, small; d = .20 or less. IPT-A = interpersonal psychotherapy for adolescents; CBT = cognitive behavior therapy; MST = multisystemic therapy; SSRI = selective serotonin reuptake inhibitor.
[a] Over 12 months. [b] See side effects and risk–benefit discussion.

with the therapist, requiring significant time and effort. In a sample of psychiatrically hospitalized adolescents, C. A. King, Hovey, Brand, Wilson, and Ghaziuddin (1997) found that youths and families were more likely to adhere to recommended psychopharmacological treatment than to recommended psychotherapy. Nevertheless, most evidence with adult patients suggests that, when given a choice, patients express a preference for psychosocial interventions over medications (Chilvers et al., 2001; Hall & Robertson, 1998; Jorm, 2000; Paykel, Hart, & Priest, 1998; Priest, Vize, Roberts, Roberts, & Tylee, 1996). There is evidence of similar preferences among youths with depression (Asarnow et al., 2003, 2005).

The absence of more substantial effect sizes for psychosocial interventions, particularly with youths experiencing suicidal tendencies or moderate or severe depression, is also a limitation. These limited effect sizes have been found despite the fact that many of the studies reported did not use intent-to-treat analyses. Furthermore, with few exceptions (e.g., Rohde et al., 2004; Rohde, Clarke, Lewinsohn, Seeley, & Kaufman, 2001), studies have not systematically examined the efficacy of psychosocial treatments for depressive disorders with such comorbid conditions as conduct disorder or alcohol and substance use disorders. The long-term effectiveness of most interventions also has not been established, and a significant proportion of youths remain depressed or only partially recovered after treatment.

Evidence for the use of these therapies in preadolescents is extremely limited. The effectiveness of IPT-A has not been studied with preadolescents and, in fact, IPT-A was named and modified specifically as a therapy for adolescents. Although CBT is generally conceptualized as a broader therapeutic approach for depression in children and adolescents, most studies of CBT targeting depression have been conducted with adolescents, including the only study of combination treatment. Stark et al. (1987) and Weisz et al. (1997) demonstrated the efficacy of group-based CBT treatment for depression in elementary school children. In general, cognitive approaches have shown no advantage over noncognitive approaches in adolescents (Weisz et al., 2006), and it is possible they will have more limited effectiveness in younger children who may not be developmentally ready to engage in challenging cognitive operations or related tasks.

Finally, limited resources may present a substantial barrier. Appropriate providers are not available in many geographic regions. Some health care insurance policies offer only limited benefits for psychosocial interventions and, more generally, for the treatment of mental health problems or psychiatric disorders, probably creating a disincentive to seek treatment.

PHARMACOLOGICAL INTERVENTIONS

Antidepressant medications are prescribed for many children and adolescents who struggle with clinical depression. Although methodological challenges and publication biases hampered early efforts to make an accurate determination of the efficacy and safety of SSRIs for children and adolescents, recent studies have provided much more information. This information has fueled a lively debate concerning the balance of risks and benefits for using these medications with youths.

Depressive Disorders

Roughly 11 million antidepressant prescriptions were written for children and adolescents in the United States during 2002 (Goode, 2004; Rigoni, 2004). Approximately 6% of outpatient physician visits for U.S. children ages 5 to 17 involved the prescription, ordering, or provision of antidepressant medication (National Center for Health Statistics, 2004). Researchers' meta-analyses have consistently indicated that tricyclics have no significant pharmacological effect on depression in children (Ambrosini, Bianchi, Rabinovich, & Elia, 1993; Dujovne, Barnard, & Rapoff, 1995; Fisher & Fisher, 1996; Hazell, O'Connell, Heathcote, Robertson, & Henry, 1995; Michael & Crowley, 2002; Sommers-Flanagan & Sommers-Flanagan, 1996). Six of the seven published randomized controlled studies of the efficacy of SSRIs in children and adolescents showed significant differences on some measures, suggesting more favorable outcomes for those treated with SSRIs (Emslie et al., 1997, 2002; Keller et al., 2001; Simeon et al., 1990; TADS, 2004; Wagner et al., 2003; Wagner, Robb, et al., 2004).

Methodological issues and publication biases have made it difficult to make an accurate determination of the efficacy of SSRIs as a treatment for children and adolescents with depressive disorders ("Depressing Research," 2004; Garland, 2004). Jureidini et al. (2004) reviewed published controlled trials of newer antidepressants in children. They found that almost half of the clinician-rated measures favored the antidepressants over placebo, but none of the patient-rated or parent-rated outcomes saw an improvement with antidepressants. In addition to questioning the clinical significance of statistically significant results, Jureidini et al. underscored the numerous methodological weaknesses of these trials, including reliance on last observation carried forward, an emphasis on secondary endpoints, transforming continuous variables into categorical outcomes (e.g., response rates) and thereby inflating small differences, and possible unblinding due to side effects from active medication. An independent analysis by the U.S. Food and Drug Administration (FDA) concluded that only 3 out of 15 randomized controlled clinical trials (including all published and unpublished datasets) of the newer antidepressants found them to be more effective than placebo on primary outcome measures in children with depression (Hammad, Laughren, & Racoosin, 2006). Several of the trials had positive and significant effects on secondary measures.

More recently, Bridge et al. (2007) conducted a review and meta-analysis of randomized placebo-controlled clinical trials assessing the use of SSRIs and other second-generation antidepressants in children and adolescents with major depressive disorder (MDD), obsessive–compulsive disorder (OCD), or non-OCD anxiety disorders. The examination of data from 13 clinical trials involving 2,910 participants indicated that positive effects of these antidepressants were modest for the treatment of MDD. The placebo response rate was 50% (95% confidence interval [CI], 47% to 53%); the antidepressant response rate was 61% (95% CI, 58% to 63%). The reported number needed to treat to benefit one youth (NNT) was 10. This meta-analysis indicates that, as a group, SSRIs and other second-generation antidepressants are associated with small positive effects for children and adolescents with MDD. As discussed further below, the analysis also indicated a risk of 1 extra suicidal patient for every 100 treated with SSRIs compared with placebo.

Suicidality

There are no published studies of psychopharmacological treatment or combined psychosocial and psychopharmacological treatment specifically targeted to suicidal youths. Youths with histories of suicide attempts, recent psychiatric hospitalizations, or substantial suicidal intent have been excluded from psychopharmacology trials, primarily because of safety concerns. The Treatment of Adolescent Suicide Attempters study, an ongoing multisite project sponsored by the National Institute of Mental Health, is collecting feasibility data (e.g., recruitment, safety monitoring, measurement procedures) in preparation for a possible definitive study addressing combination treatments for suicidal youths with depressive disorders.

Strength of Evidence

The FDA identified 15 controlled studies of antidepressants in children, but only 3 resulted in an advantage of the antidepressant over inert placebo. The FDA did not count the additional TADS study as a positive study for SSRIs as a singular treatment because of the negative findings for the Children's Depression Rating Scale—Revised (Kovacs, 2003), which was the primary depression outcome measure. The methodology appears sound, but the evidence base in support of antidepressants in children is relatively weak. The placebo-related effects account for the majority of variance in children's outcomes.

Concerns have been raised about the safety of SSRIs as a treatment for children and adolescents. The FDA conducted a meta-analysis of 24 placebo-controlled trials (published and unpublished), which included more than 4,400 youth participants (Hammad, Laughren, & Racoosin, 2006). Their data indicated that antidepressant medications were associated with a doubling of the risk for suicidal behavior or suicidal ideation, relative to placebo, although the absolute risk was small (4% vs. 2%) and no suicides were reported. A more recent meta-analysis reported that the absolute rates of suicidal ideation and attempts were 3% in participants receiving antidepressants and 2% in those receiving placebo (Bridge et al., 2007). Findings are consistent, albeit slightly different, as this meta-analysis included additional studies and used a different data analytic strategy than that used by the FDA. Finally, Olfson, Marcus, and Shaffer (2006) used a matched case-control design to estimate the relative risk of suicide attempt and suicide in severely depressed children and adults treated with versus without antidepressant medication. These were Medicaid beneficiaries who had received inpatient treatment for depression. Olfson et al. reported small significant relationships between antidepressant treatment and both suicide attempts and deaths in children and adolescents.

In 2004, the FDA issued a black box warning label requirement for antidepressant medications, indicating that they increased the risk of suicidal ideation and behavior in some children and adolescents. More recently, this black box warning has been extended to include young adults. The content of this warning is as follows (FDA, 2007):

> Suicidality and Antidepressant Drugs
>
> Antidepressants increased the risk compared to placebo of suicidal thinking and behavior (suicidality) in children, adolescents, and young adults in short-term studies of major depressive disorder (MDD) and other psychiatric disorders. Anyone considering the use of [Insert established name] or any other antidepressant in a child, adolescent, or young adult must balance this risk with the clinical need. Short-term studies did not show an increase in the risk of suicidality with antidepressants compared to placebo in adults beyond age 24; there was a reduction in risk with antidepressants compared to placebo in adults aged 65 and older. Depression and certain other psychiatric disorders are themselves associated with increases in the risk of suicide. Patients of all ages who are started on antidepressant therapy should be monitored appropriately and observed closely for clinical worsening, suicidality, or unusual changes in behavior. Families and caregivers should be advised of the need for close observation and communication with the prescriber. [Insert Drug Name] is not approved for use in pediatric patients. [The previous sentence would be replaced with the sentence, below, for the following drugs: Prozac: Prozac is approved for use in pediatric patients with MDD and obsessive compulsive disorder (OCD). Zoloft: Zoloft is not approved for use in pediatric patients except for patients with obsessive compulsive disorder (OCD). Fluvoxamine: Fluvoxamine is not approved for use in pediatric patients except for patients with obsessive compulsive disorder (OCD).] (See Warnings: Clinical Worsening and Suicide Risk, Precautions: Information for Patients, and Precautions: Pediatric Use)

Side Effects

Knowledge of side-effect profiles is based primarily on studies involving adults. The most common side effects of SSRIs in studies of patients with depressive disorders include agitation, sleep disruption, gastrointestinal symptoms, and sexual problems (Antonuccio, Danton, DeNelsky, Greenberg, & Gordon, 1999). Evidence from animal studies indicates that SSRIs may cause gonadal tissue shrinkage (U.S. Department of Health & Human Services, 2004), and recent case reports in adults suggest that sexual side effects may persist in a small minority of cases even after medication is withdrawn (Csoka & Shipko, 2006). These data, along with case reports of growth suppression in children that may be linked to SSRIs (Weintrob, Cohen, Klipper-Aurbach, Zadik, & Dickerman, 2002), raise concerns about the possibility that antidepressants could alter the course of pubertal growth and development in adolescents. Even though this has not been systematically investigated to date, the consequences are dire enough to warrant utmost caution and mandate immediate research.

Side effects and medical risks increase when SSRIs are combined with other medications (Antonuccio et al., 1999; Dalfen & Stewart, 2001). In addition, the withdrawal symptoms of SSRIs are substantial for many patients (Coupland, Bell, & Potokar, 1996; Fava, 2002; Rosenbaum, Fava, Hoog, Ashcroft, & Krebs, 1998). Increased risk for manic episodes (e.g., Preda, MacLean, Mazure, & Bowers, 2001) and acts of deliberate self-harm (e.g., Donovan et al., 2000; Healy, 2003) are a critical cause for concern. Although the data are mixed and somewhat controversial, other potential risks that warrant further investigation include the association of antidepressants with breast cancer (e.g., Bahl, Cotterchio, & Kreiger, 2003; Cotterchio, Kreiger, Darlington, & Steingart, 2000; Halbreich, Shen, & Panaro, 1996; Moorman, Grubber, Millikan, & Newman, 2003; Sharpe, Collet, Belzile, Hanley, & Boivin, 2002) and the possibility of irreversible biochemical changes predisposing some susceptible patients to chronic depression (e.g., Ansorge, Zhou, Lira, Hen, & Gingrich, 2004; Baldessarini, 1995; Fava, 1995, 2002). As noted in chapter 6 on anxiety disorders, the only SSRI that is approved by the FDA for use in the pediatric population is fluoxetine.

COMBINED INTERVENTIONS

TADS (2004) enrolled 439 patients between the ages of 12 and 17 years with sustained (i.e., at least 6 weeks) and moderately severe or severe major depression. These adolescents were randomly assigned to 12 weeks of the SSRI fluoxetine alone, CBT alone, CBT combined with fluoxetine, or placebo. The variant of CBT used in this study consisted of individual therapy, psychoeducation, and conjoint parent–adolescent sessions. Combining various cognitive and behavioral strategies was more comprehensive and modular, with less time spent on cognitive restructuring, than the CBT used in Brent et al.'s (1997) study. On the primary depression endpoint (the Children's Depression Rating Scale—Revised; Kovacs, 2003), combined treatment was superior to other treatment conditions, whereas neither fluoxetine alone nor CBT alone separated from placebo.

Response rates on a global improvement measure in the TADS (2004) study were 71% for the combined treatment, 61% for fluoxetine alone, 43% for CBT alone, and 35% for placebo, with the two fluoxetine-containing conditions superior to CBT and to placebo but also resulting in twice as many harm-related adverse side effects. The pattern of findings suggested that CBT has a small protective effect on suicidality, with CBT alone resulting in the lowest rate of harm-related side effects (4.5%), fluoxetine alone having the highest (11.9%), and the combination in the middle (8.4%). This may reflect the benefit of learning coping skills in the CBT conditions. A conservative treatment strategy designed to minimize risk might involve a sequential approach using psychosocial interventions initially, close monitoring, and the addition of fluoxetine for nonresponders whose parents are fully informed of the potential risks and benefits.

It will be extremely important to examine longer term follow-up findings as to safety issues and the differential (and combined) efficacy of CBT and fluoxetine. This is critical given that the most suicidal youths were excluded from the TADS study (i.e., those with suicidal intent, a suicide attempt requiring medical attention within the past 6 months, or suicidal ideation with disorganized family). That is, there is a lack of safety data concerning the use of antidepressants with a more fully representative sample (and indeed, the most critical sample) of adolescents with depression. Examination of the possible long-term protective effect of CBT is also crucial. Studies have found that adults treated to remission with CBT are significantly less likely to relapse following treatment termination than adults treated to remission with medications alone (Hollon et al., 2005), although so far there is no indication of this in studies with children (Birmaher et al., 2000; Brent et al., 1999).

Strength of Evidence

There has been one scientifically rigorous, multisite, randomized controlled clinical trial assessing efficacy and safety outcomes associated with fluoxetine alone, CBT alone, CBT in combination with fluoxetine, or placebo in adolescents. Combination treatment was superior to other treatment conditions, the two medication conditions were superior to CBT and to placebo (but also associated with twice as many harm-related adverse side effects), and CBT had a small protective effect on suicidality. Replication of these findings will be important. In addition, evidence concerning the longer-term efficacy (including the impact on adaptive functioning) and safety outcomes is needed. Some of this evidence will be forthcoming from the TADS trial. A preliminary efficacy analysis suggests that CBT alone caught up with fluoxetine alone at 18-week follow-up and CBT alone caught up with the combined condition by 36-week follow-up (Kuehn, 2007).

Limitations

Despite the fact that combination treatment has shown greater efficacy than either antidepressants or CBT alone in the short-term treatment of moderate to severe MDD in adolescents, such treatment will not always be available to families. Furthermore, some families may prefer to begin treatment with a psychosocial treatment or placebo approach because of concerns about even the small increases in adverse events that have been associated with medication. Other families may prefer medication over the time and effort (and other resources) involved in participating in regularly scheduled psychotherapy. It should be noted that there is no evidence for the efficacy and safety of combination treatment relative to singular treatments in preadolescents.

DIVERSITY

Studies on depression treatment have not generally examined the extent to which age, gender, race, and ethnicity moderate the efficacy of psychosocial interventions and pharmacotherapy for children and adolescents with depressive disorders. In fact, this has not even been a possibility in most studies because of small sample sizes or samples that lacked sufficient variability for such analyses. For instance, many studies on depression include samples that are predominantly female (e.g., Rosselló & Bernal, 1999), raising questions about the generalizability of results to males. Most studies have limited recruitment to either preadolescents (e.g., Stark et al., 1987; Weisz et al., 1997) or adolescents (e.g., Lewinsohn et al., 1990; Reynolds & Coats, 1986; TADS, 2004), making it impossible to examine whether age group (preadolescent vs. adolescent) moderates treatment efficacy. This lack of diverse participants is being rectified to some extent by the TADS study, in which moderator analyses are being conducted.

Finally, most depression treatment studies have sampled primarily White or, in the case of IPT, Hispanic populations, but no depression treatment studies have reported efficacy for specific racial or ethnic groups. This is the case despite evidence that drug adherence and metabolism are affected by ethnocultural issues (Lin, Poland, & Nakasaki, 1993; C. Muñoz & Hilgenberg, 2005; R. F. Muñoz, Hollon, McGrath, Rehm, & VandenBos, 1994) and that minorities are much less likely to seek mental health treatment than those from the majority culture (C. Muñoz & Hilgenberg, 2005). Thus, existing knowledge of evidence-based treatments is only general when the population in need is very diverse. Further research examining treatment effects and outcomes by diversity variables is necessary. It will be important to learn what treatments are efficacious for specific populations of youths. Equally important will be to train providers to implement these treatments in a culturally and linguistically competent manner so that minorities can make better use of the broader range of options beyond psychopharmacology.

RISK–BENEFIT ANALYSIS

The acceptability of the risk–benefit profile with fluoxetine, the only antidepressant to show consistent evidence of some benefit in children with depression and the only SSRI approved by the FDA for use with children and adolescents, involves value judgments as to the cost of harm-related and psychiatric-related adverse side effects. The risk of increased suicidality appears to be relatively low (i.e., 2 suicidal patients for every 100 treated with an SSRI compared with a placebo), and no patients actually completed suicide in the FDA database of controlled trials, but the stakes are clearly high. Furthermore, because randomized trials involving antidepressants have excluded suicidal patients, data concerning potential risk are limited and, indeed, have not focused on the youths most at risk.

Whittington et al. (2004) reviewed the available data (published and unpublished) from controlled trials of SSRIs in youths with depressive disorders. Their meta-analysis showed that the risk–benefit profile (number needed to treat to benefit one extra patient [NNTB] vs. number needed to treat before a serious adverse harm event happened to one extra patient [NNTH]) was favorable for fluoxetine but was unfavorable for paroxetine, sertraline, citalopram, and venlafaxine because of poor efficacy and increased risk of harm-related behaviors.

The TADS (2004) study, conducted more recently than the studies included in the review by Whittington et al. (2004), offers the only data pertinent to the short-term relative risks of offering patients psychotherapy alone, medication alone, the combination, or a placebo. Despite the fact that suicidality decreased across all four arms of this study, fluoxetine was associated with a significantly higher rate of harm-related side effects (such as suicidal ideation), physiological side effects (diarrhea, insomnia, and sedation), and psychiatric side effects (irritability, mania, and fatigue) compared with placebo or CBT alone. Using the global response rate outcome from the TADS study, the NNTB is about 3 in the combined condition, 5 for fluoxetine alone, and 12 for CBT alone, all compared with placebo.

In terms of harm-related adverse side effects, the NNTH is approximately 20 in the fluoxetine-containing conditions compared with the nonmedication conditions. Considering psychiatric-related adverse side effects, the NNTH is approximately 10 in the fluoxetine-alone condition compared with placebo and only about 5 compared with CBT alone. Trade-offs like these have led regulatory bodies in Europe, Britain, Canada, Australia, and the United States to issue stern warnings or outright contraindications for the use of antidepressants in children. When risk of harm is considered in a cost–benefit analysis together with medical cost offset (Hunsley, 2003), relapse, and side effects, psychological interventions can be very cost-effective (Antonuccio, Thomas, & Danton, 1997). These drugs generally have modest side effects in the short term, but they can also have extremely serious side effects. Also, their long-term effects on the central nervous system of children and adolescents are still unknown, making this work crucial in future research.

FUTURE DIRECTIONS

Clinical depression has an indisputably adverse impact on the development trajectories of children and adolescents. Despite this well-established fact and the recent increase in depression treatment research, the evidence for a singular treatment approach involving antidepressant medication or CBT suggests only modest positive effects achieved with a substantial investment of resources. The specific advantages over placebo for either treatment alone have been modest in many studies and nonexistent in some studies. One large-scale study does, however, suggest that a combined treatment may be more effective in the short term (TADS, 2004). It is clear that clinical scientists have only moved a short way toward the goal of developing evidence-based interventions that reduce depression severity and its associated functional impairment and, ultimately, enable children and adolescents to achieve sustained depression recovery. Additional research is needed to improve the efficacy and safety of existing psychopharmacological and psychosocial interventions, to replicate findings concerning the efficacy of IPT with independent teams of investigators, to consider other theoretically based interventions, and to continue to examine the potential benefit of combined treatments. Additional research efforts are also needed to investigate the long-term safety and efficacy for children and adolescents.

Studies of the comparative efficacy of psychosocial and pharmacological interventions are less common in children than in adults, and available evidence leaves open the question of whether their short-term efficacy differs in a clinically meaningful way. The TADS (2004) study found no differences between singular treatments on the primary depression outcome measure; however, there was greater improvement with SSRI treatment on a secondary measure. In contrast, available evidence seems to suggest a short-term risk advantage for psychosocial interventions, although harm has only recently been systematically and carefully evaluated. In summary, the benefits and risks of various treatment options or combined treatments must be weighed against the benefits and risks of providing no or inadequate treatment for depression, a condition that is associated with substantial morbidity, mortality, and reduced quality of life (Brent, 2004).

It is striking how little is known about even some of the most basic issues of depression in youths. Additional studies are needed to determine the efficacy of these treatments in younger children, the mechanisms of action in CBT and IPT psychotherapies, the long-term benefits and risks of individual and combined treatments, the safest and most efficacious sequencing of psychosocial and psychopharmacological treatments, the potential differential efficacy of treatments for boys and girls and different racial and ethnic groups, and the extent to which treatments are beneficial in depressed youths with comorbid psychiatric disorders. Particularly striking is that almost all available data from clinical trials pertain to adolescents.

It is ironic that the specific advantages of available treatments for youths with depression, whether psychosocial or psychopharmacological, are small compared with the nonspecific effects of placebo and other supportive comparison treatments. It could be argued that more resources are warranted to investigate and train practitioners in the nonspecifics of the therapeutic alliance, support, exposure, and problem-solving skills that seem to cut across many treatments. It could also be argued that watchful waiting may be appropriate for some youths who exhibit milder symptoms of depression.

Data to guide the treatment of suicidal youths are even more limited. In addition to highlighting the importance of additional focused research in this area, studies conducted thus far suggest that multilayered or sequenced interventions may be needed to intervene effectively with suicidal youths (C. A. King et al., 2006). It will be important to address the diagnostic heterogeneity that characterizes these youths and to target the chronic psychopathology and psychosocial difficulties that are often present.

8

BIPOLAR DISORDER

The diagnosis of *bipolar disorder* (BPD) in children has been controversial. In particular, the core symptoms necessary for diagnosis, the necessity of discrete episodes, and the definitions of cycling have been debated, and their application is not consistent across studies (Kowatch & Fristad, 2006). *Classic Bipolar I disorder* is not common in youths; *bipolar spectrum disorders* (Bipolar I, mania plus depression; Bipolar II, hypomania plus depression; cyclothymia, hypomania plus "hypodepression" [i.e., subsyndromal depression]; and *bipolar disorder not otherwise specified* [BPD-NOS]) are common (Kowatch & Fristad, 2006). When BPD-NOS is diagnosed, the reason for this diagnosis should be stated clearly and specifically (e.g., one symptom below threshold, duration less than 7 days). In all cases, careful observation of children and receipt of information from multiple informants are important.

The diagnostic criteria for a manic episode require "a distinct period of abnormally and persistently elevated, expansive, or irritable mood, lasting at least 1 week" (American Psychiatric Association, 2000, p. 332). However, irritability is pervasive in childhood disorders, so some clinical researchers have required hallmark criteria of expansive or elated mood or grandiosity before diagnosing mania in children (D. A. Geller et al., 2000). Additionally, many children meet symptom criteria for mania, with the exception of the duration criterion. These children may have intense rapid mood swings and are often diagnosed with BPD-NOS.

In BPD diagnosis, developmental issues must be constantly considered. Because cognitive maturation influences children's experience of and expression of emotional states, children may be less able to express symptoms such as hopelessness, and their limited ability to compare and evaluate themselves against others makes low self-esteem more difficult to assess (Klaus & Fristad, in press). Additionally, the expression of manic symptoms such as grandiosity, increased goal-directed activity, and excessive involvement in pleasurable activities varies on the basis of age and must be differentiated from typical childhood behaviors. Use of frequency, intensity, number, and duration of symptoms criteria, sometimes called FIND (Kowatch et al., 2005), can assist the clinician in determining when a behavior is a symptom and not merely a manifestation of ordinary developmental differences or stages.

More recently, with phenomenological studies shedding light on course of illness (B. Geller et al., 2000, 2001, 2002; B. Geller, Tillman, Craney, & Bolhofner, 2004), empirical guidelines for the diagnosis of Bipolar I have improved, although less examination of the diagnostic boundaries for Bipolar II, BPD-NOS, and cyclothymia has occurred (Kowatch et al., 2005). The National Institute of Mental Health (NIMH) recently funded a four-site study, the Longitudinal Assessment of Manic Symptoms, that should lend clarity to diagnostic parameters for these bipolar spectrum disorders. These diagnoses can be made in preschool children (Tumuluru, Weller, Fristad, & Weller, 2003; Wilens et al., 2003) but should be done cautiously.

As with depression, earlier age of onset appears to be associated with a stronger genetic loading and a more pernicious course, although data on preschool children with BPD are limited (Kowatch & Fristad, 2006). Relatively little is known about prevalence rates. Lewinsohn, Seeley, and Klein (1995) reported lifetime prevalence rates of 1% for the diagnosis of BPD, with an additional 5.7% with subthreshold symptoms. These adolescents experienced functional impairments similar to the BPD group into young adulthood. However, this study was based solely on interviews with adolescents, and more recent research has emphasized the importance of including parent report in diagnosing BPD (Youngstrom et al., 2004). Particular attention should be paid to issues of differential diagnosis and comorbidity, because the overlap of symptoms found in attention-deficit/hyperactivity disorder, posttraumatic stress disorder, and BPD is significant.

PSYCHOSOCIAL INTERVENTIONS

Three research groups have tested psychosocial interventions for BPD. All or most participants in psychosocial treatment studies were on concomitant medication, consistent with current treatment guidelines (Kowatch et al., 2005). Pavuluri et al. (2004) reported that 34 youths ages 5 to 18, nonrandomly assigned to the RAINBOW psychosocial program in a specialty medication clinic, fared better at follow-up than those managed with standard clinic care. Miklowitz et al. (2004) provided adjunctive family-focused psychoeducational treatment to 20 youths ages 13 to 18 years in an open trial and noted improvement in depressive, manic, and behavioral symptoms over a 1-year follow-up. Miklowitz et al. continue to pilot a randomized clinical trial for adolescents with BPD. Fristad et al. conducted three randomized clinical trials, two with multifamily psychoeducation groups and one with individual family psychoeducation (Fristad, Gavazzi, & Mackinaw-Koons, 2003; Fristad, Goldberg-Arnold, & Gavazzi, 2002, 2003). All three trials indicated that children ages 8 to 12 and their families demonstrated improvement across a variety of symptom and functional outcome measures following brief, structured intervention. Table 8.1 provides a summary of treatment efficacy for bipolar disorders.

Strength of Evidence

Despite limited data, interventions used by the investigators previously described have more similarities than differences in their content. Results across studies are comparable, lending support to the concept that psychoeducationally oriented interventions are effective adjunctive treatments in the comprehensive care of children and adolescents with BPD.

Limitations

There are too few published studies to define limitations. Only four randomized clinical trials have been conducted, and only two of these are completed. The other two are nearing completion. Three of the four trials were pilot studies with small sample sizes. Only one study is with adolescents; three are with children ages 8 to 12.

PHARMACOLOGICAL INTERVENTIONS

Few randomized double-blind psychopharmacological studies for BPD have been conducted, but treatment guidelines based on combining available evidence with expert opinion have recently been published (Kowatch et al., 2005). These guidelines list evidence for the treatment of Bipolar I with psychosis, Bipolar I without psychosis, and BPD-depressed episode. A review was conducted to determine whether articles had been published since the guidelines went into press. Ten additional articles were found; none added incremental evidence.

TABLE 8.1
Treatment Efficacy for Bipolar Disorder

Treatment	Acute		Long term[a]		Side effects[b]
	Strength of evidence and effect size, Primary symptoms	Strength of evidence and effect size, Functional outcomes	Strength of evidence and effect size, Primary symptoms	Strength of evidence and effect size, Functional outcomes	
Psychosocial					
CFF–CBT	4a, Mania, depression, ADHD, psychosis, aggression, and sleep disturbances	4a, Overall functioning	No data	No data	None reported
FFT	4b, Symptoms of depression and mania 4a, Internalizing and externalizing symptoms	No data	No data	No data	None reported
MFPG	No data	2a, Parents' knowledge of mood disorders 2c, Positive expressed emotion 2b, Negative expressed emotion	No data	No data	None reported
IFP	2b, Mood severity	No data	No data	No data	None reported

Medication					
Lithium	2a, Symptoms of mania 4a, Symptoms of depression, symptoms of mania, psychotic symptoms, and overall psychiatric illness 4b, Symptoms of mania, symptoms of depression, and psychotic symptoms	4a, Overall functioning	No data	No data	Weight gain, polydipsia, polyuria, headache, tremor, gastrointestinal pain, nausea, vomiting, anorexia, diarrhea, hypothyroidism.
Carbamazepine	2a, Symptoms of mania	No data	No data	No data	Nausea but most side effects mild to moderate and tolerated by most participants, risk for neutropenia, agranulocytopenia, thrombocytopenia.
Divalproex sodium	2a, Symptoms of mania, symptoms of depression, and psychotic symptoms 4a, Symptoms of mania, symptoms of depression, and aggression 4b, Psychotic symptoms	4a, Overall functioning	No data	No data	Risk for liver toxicity, liver failure, pancreatitis, weight gain, polycystic ovary syndrome.
Topiramate	4a, Overall psychiatric illness and symptoms of mania 2b, Symptoms of mania	4a, Overall functioning	No data	No data	Diarrhea, somnolence
Quetiapine	2a, Symptoms of mania, symptoms of depression, and psychotic symptoms	No data	No data	No data	Sedation, dizziness, gastrointestinal upset
Olanzapine	4a, Symptoms of mania 2a, Symptoms of mania 2b, Psychotic symptoms, and symptoms of depression	No data	No data	No data	Cognitive disturbance, dysphoria, gastrointestinal disturbances, tremors, sedation, blurry vision.

(continues)

TABLE 8.1
(Continued)

Treatment	Acute: Strength of evidence and effect size, Primary symptoms	Acute: Strength of evidence and effect size, Functional outcomes	Long term[a]: Strength of evidence and effect size, Primary symptoms	Long term[a]: Strength of evidence and effect size, Functional outcomes	Side effects[b]
Risperidone	4a, Symptoms of mania, aggression, psychotic symptoms, ADHD symptoms, and symptoms of depression 2a, Symptom of mania, psychotic symptoms, and symptoms of depression	No data	No data	No data	Increased appetite, somnolence, abdominal pain, weight gain.
Combination					
Lithium + adjunctive psychotic	4a, Symptoms of mania, symptoms of depression, psychotic symptoms, and overall psychiatric illness	4a, Overall functioning	No data	No data	None reported
Divalproex sodium + risperidone	2a, Symptoms of mania, symptoms of depression, aggression, and psychotic symptoms	2a, Overall functioning	No data	No data	Weight gain, sedation, nausea, increased appetite, stomach pain, tremors, cognitive dulling, akathisia, galactorrhea.
Lithium + risperidone	2a, Symptoms of mania, symptoms of depression, and aggression 2b, Psychotic symptoms	2a, Overall functioning	No data	No data	Weight gain, sedation, nausea, increased appetite, stomach pain, tremors, cognitive dulling, akathisia, polyuria, buccolingual movements.

Lithium + divalproex sodium	4a, Symptoms of mania, symptoms of depression, overall psychiatric illness	4a, Overall functioning	No data	No data	Emesis, enuresis, stomach pain, tremor, increased thirst, headache, nausea, sedation, increased appetite, diarrhea, decreased appetite, respiratory congestion, fever with flue symptoms, dizziness, body ache.
Divalproex sodium + quetiapine	2b, Symptoms of mania	No data	No data	No data	Sedation, nausea, headache, and gastrointestinal irritation.

Note. Across all treatment studies for each type of child psychopathology, we used guidelines put forth by J. Cohen (1988): Strength of evidence: 1 = replicated clinical trial or large-body, single-subject study; 2 = controlled clinical trial or replicated, single-subject study; 3 = comparison group but not clinical trial; 4 = no control group. Effect size: a = .81+, large; b = .51 to .80, medium; c = .21 to .50, small; d = .20 or less. CFF–CBT = child and family-focused cognitive behavior therapy; FFT = family focused therapy; MFPG = multifamily psychoeducation groups; IFP = individual family psychoeducation.
[a]Over 12 months. [b]See side effects and risk–benefit discussion.

Strength of Evidence

Lithium is the best-studied medication for BPD, with evidence supporting its use. Even the randomized controlled trials, however, have limitations like small sample size and methodological issues, including crossover designs, that are less than ideal for a cyclic disorder (Kowatch et al., 2005). Open trials also support use of lithium (Kafantaris, Coletti, Dicker, Padula, & Kane, 2001, 2003). Quetiapine was effective in a double-blind, placebo-control trial as an adjunct to valproate (Del Bello, Schwiers, Rosenberg, & Strakowski, 2002). A multicenter trial funded by the NIMH is currently under way to determine the efficacy of lithium in children with Bipolar I. Another study of lithium pharmacokinetics, efficacy, safety, and effectiveness is beginning under a contract by the National Institute of Child Health and Human Development. A large, multisite trial funded by NIMH is in progress to compare the relative effectiveness of lithium, valproate, and risperidone in children ages 8 to 14 with Bipolar I.

Open trials, with methodological limitations, also support the use of divalproex (Kowatch et al., 2000; Papatheodorou & Kutcher, 1993; Papatheodorou, Kutcher, Katic, & Szalai, 1995; Wagner et al., 2002; West et al., 1994, 1995), clozapine (Kowatch et al., 1995), carbamazepine (Kowatch et al., 2000), olanzapine (Frazier et al., 2001), and topirimate as an adjunctive intervention (Del Bello et al., 2002). There is retrospective evidence for the efficacy of risperidone (Frazier et al., 1999). Limited studies are available for BPD-depressed episode. No randomized controlled trials have been conducted with youths. Investigators conducting open trials, reviewing charts, and reporting cases suggest that divalproex (Kowatch et al., 2000), lamotrigine (Kusumaker & Yatham, 1997), and selective serotonin reuptake inhibitors (SSRIs; Biederman, Lopez, Boellner, & Chandler, 2002) are beneficial, but SSRIs have also been known to result in an unstable mood.

Side Effects

Side effects associated with psychotropic medication for BPD are common and range from nuisance to more severe toxicities. Some medications, such as atypical antipsychotics, can induce weight gain, which can result in a series of general metabolic disorders, including Type 2 (noninsulin-dependent) diabetes mellitus, lipid level changes, and transaminase elevation (Kowatch et al., 2005). The American Diabetes Association, in conjunction with the American Psychiatric Association, American Association of Clinical Endocrinologists, and North American Association for the Study of Obesity (2004), published a monitoring protocol for all individuals receiving atypical antipsychotic medications. There are anecdotal reports of adverse cognitive side effects from essentially all medications used for mood stabilization, including problems with word retrieval, working memory, and cognitive dulling. Polycystic ovarian syndrome is related to the use of divalproex in women. Current guidelines suggest monitoring menstrual patterns as well as weight gain in women prescribed divalproex (Kowatch et al., 2005).

Medications and other uncommon but problematic side effects that warrant monitoring include lithium (hypothyroidism), antipsychotics (abnormal involuntary movements, prolactin elevation), divalproex (pancreatitis), ziprasidone (intracardiac conduction effects), and clozapine (hematological and neurological adverse events and neuroleptic malignant syndrome).

COMBINED INTERVENTIONS

Essentially no psychosocial trials have occurred in the absence of concomitant pharmacotherapy, and no medication studies for BPD have tested the adjunctive benefit of psychosocial intervention. Studies that include both medication and therapy have not used a dismantling methodology to determine the unique contribution of each treatment. Thus, no empirical guidelines on the incremental benefit of concomitant medication and therapy have been established.

DIVERSITY

Treatment studies have been too small in size for any meaningful comparisons to be made between treatment response for boys versus girls, or minority versus majority racial or ethnic groups. Biederman et al. (2004) examined 74 girls and 224 boys from their outpatient clinic, all of whom met criteria for BPD (American Psychiatric Association, 2000). They found no meaningful differences in symptom expression, types of treatment received, severity of educational deficits, severity of family and interpersonal functioning, or patterns of comorbidity between boys and girls. Further research examining treatment effects and outcomes by diversity variables is necessary.

RISK–BENEFIT ANALYSIS

There are few long-term safety studies conducted for many of the medications used to treat BPD, and of those available, most are with adult participants. It is critical for clinicians, youths, and parents to consider a risk–benefit analysis when determining what medications to try in the treatment of BPD. Psychosocial interventions seem to confer benefit with no risk; thus, psychosocial treatment of BPD is advised. Psychotropic agents are considered first-line treatment in all published treatment guidelines (Kowatch et al., 2005). Unfortunately, they can bring significant risk. Many more clinical trials in children are needed to examine the efficacy and safety of these medications. The development of safe and effective psychotropic agents to manage BPD in children is sorely needed.

FUTURE DIRECTIONS

Nonpharmacological physiologic interventions have not been tested in children and adolescents with bipolar spectrum disorders. However, a rationale for testing several interventions has been provided by adult studies, including vagus nerve stimulation and transcranial magnetic stimulation (Hirshberg, Chiu, & Frazier, 2005).

Two consensus statements emphasize the need for pharmacological and psychosocial management of BPD (Coyle et al., 2003; Kowatch et al., 2005), but studies designed to test the relative contribution of both treatment components have not been conducted. There is growing agreement over the diagnosis of Bipolar I in youths, but there is less clarity about the clinical profiles of youths with bipolar spectrum disorders (Bipolar II, cyclothymia, and BPD-NOS). Unfortunately, research on pharmacological and psychosocial interventions for BPD is lacking, and empirical guidelines for their combination are also lacking. Currently, clinical guidelines exist for the assessment and treatment of BPD in youths (Kowatch et al., 2005); it is anticipated these will be modified as new research is completed. A multisite research study to address this has begun.

9

SCHIZOPHRENIA SPECTRUM DISORDERS

Psychosis can occur across a range of disorders appearing in childhood. For example, when psychotic or psychotic-like symptoms occur during the severe manifestation of obsessive–compulsive disorder, posttraumatic stress disorder, major depressive disorder, or bipolar disorder, they are considered evidence of the severity of that condition rather than an indicator of a separate diagnostic condition. Schizophrenia spectrum conditions, per se, are rare in childhood, although diagnostic procedures are well defined for children age 8 and older (Asarnow, Tompson, & McGrath, 2004). Thomsen (1996) examined all youths hospitalized for schizophrenia over a 13-year period in Denmark. Of 312 patients, only 1% had onset prior to age 13 and only 9% prior to age 15. Boys are twice as likely as girls to be diagnosed before age 18 (McClellan, Werry, & Work Group on Quality Issues, 2001). Early onset is associated with poorer outcome and higher rates of negative symptoms in adulthood (McClellan et al., 2001).

Premorbid abnormalities are common and include social withdrawal, isolation, disruptive behavior disorders, academic difficulties, speech and language problems, and developmental delays (McClellan et al., 2001). Symptoms tend to shift over time from positive (i.e., hallucinations, delusions, disorganized speech, and behavior) to negative (i.e., flat affect, anergia, social withdrawal). McClellan et al. found 10% to 20% of youths with the disorder have IQs in the borderline range or below.

Most youths with *schizophrenia spectrum disorders* maintain these diagnoses over time (Asarnow et al., 2004). Variable functional outcome has been reported. Werry, McClellan, and Chard (1991) reported the worst findings, with only 17% of their sample in school or employed full time 1 to 16 years (5 years, on average) after study entry. In a longer follow-up (6–40 years, with 16 years on average), Eggers, Bunk, and Ropcke (2002) reported only 7% of their sample to be in stable partnerships, although 73% were involved in some type of employment. Asarnow and Tompson (1999) followed a cohort of youths for 3 to 7 years following diagnosis and reported 56% had improvement in functioning, with 28% reporting relatively good psychosocial adjustment (Global Assessment of Functioning scores $\geq$ 60).

Because of the low prevalence rate, little is known about schizophrenia spectrum disorders in youths. Most of what is known about psychosocial and psychopharmacological treatment comes from studies of adults. This seems hardly satisfactory considering the vast physiological and psychological differences between adults and youths.

PSYCHOSOCIAL INTERVENTIONS

Asarnow et al. (2004) conducted meta-analyses of adult studies and found that family psychoeducation and cognitive behavior therapy can help reduce relapse, with weaker support for social skills training and no evidence of efficacy for cognitive remediation. A review of studies examining psychosocial treatment for first-episode psychosis comes to similar conclusions (Penn, Waldheter, Perkins, Mueser, & Lieberman, 2005). Of note, four recently conducted comprehensive studies were reviewed, but few participants in these studies were under age 18. Three of the four studies included participants under age 18, but most participants in each study were over age 18. This is consistent with data indicating schizophrenia onset typically ranges from ages 16 to 30 (Mueser & McGurk, 2004). One study examined 12 adolescents with schizophrenia treated over a 2-year period. Treatment was a comprehensive program that included hospitalization ranging from several months to 1 year and an intensive outpatient psychoeducational program that began upon discharge. These 12 were compared with 12 historical control participants from the same setting who received an unspecified combination of individual psychotherapy, neuroleptic medication, and milieu therapy while hospitalized. The experimental group was less likely than the control group to experience two or more hospitalizations, and their degree of improvement in psychosocial functioning was greater. Additionally, their cost of care was lower in the 2-year period than that of the control group.

Family involvement in treatment may be especially important in treating children, who developmentally are more dependent on family members. In particular, the role of *expressed emotion* (EE, an interaction style characterized by critical, hostile, intrusive interchanges) seems important for treatment. In Butzlaff and Hooley's (1998) meta-analysis of studies examining EE in adults, 65% of patients returning to homes characterized as high in EE relapsed within 1 year compared with 35% who returned to homes low in EE.

A case study of a 9-year-old with *schizoaffective disorder* described improved functioning following an eight-session multifamily psychoeducational group intervention for children with mood disorders (Klaus, Fristad, Malkin, & Koons, 2005). A randomized study of 97 families having a family member age 16 to 26 with schizophrenia indicated that those receiving family intervention in addition to standard intervention spent an average of 10 months less in institutional care at a 5-year follow-up (Lenior, Dingemans, Linszen, de Haan, & Schene, 2001). Community-based maintenance is clearly associated with improved functional outcome for adults (Simmonds, Coid, Joseph, Marriott, & Tyler, 2001), with similar results reported for children with serious emotional disturbance, not all of whom had a diagnosis of psychosis (Henggeler, Schoenwald, Rowland, & Cunningham, 2002). Table 9.1 provides a summary of treatment efficacy for schizophrenia spectrum disorders.

Strength of Evidence

Due to data from controlled investigations, the strength of the evidence is at this time limited to uncontrolled case reports.

Limitations

There are no clinical trials of psychosocial interventions on children to report. There is one historical control study of adolescents suggesting that psychoeducationally oriented comprehensive care is beneficial. Adult studies and case reports suggest psychosocial intervention is an important adjunct in the treatment of schizophrenia spectrum disorders.

PHARMACOLOGICAL INTERVENTIONS

In adults, antipsychotic medication is considered the sine qua non of treatment (Mueser & McGurk, 2004). A study conducted by Harrigan, McGorry, and Hrstev (2003) indicated that the duration of untreated psychosis is an independent predictor of poor outcome in adults, suggesting the importance of rapid intervention when psychotic symptoms emerge.

In both adults and children, traditional neuroleptics and atypical antipsychotic agents are considered first-line agents (McClellan et al., 2001;

TABLE 9.1
Treatment Efficacy for Schizophrenia Spectrum Disorders

Treatment	Acute		Long term[a]		Side effects[b]
	Strength of evidence and effect size, Primary symptoms	Strength of evidence and effect size, Functional outcomes	Strength of evidence and effect size, Primary symptoms	Strength of evidence and effect size, Functional outcomes	
Medication					
Haloperidol	2c, Hallucinations, delusions	No data	No data	No data	Mild to moderate sedation, extrapyramidal symptoms.
Risperidone	2c, Hallucinations, delusions	No data	No data	No data	Mild to moderate sedation, extrapyramidal symptoms, weight gain, metabolic syndrome.
Olanzapine	2c, Hallucinations, delusions	No data	No data	No data	Mild to moderate sedation, weight gain, metabolic syndrome.
Clozapine	2c, Hallucinations, delusions, negative symptoms	No data	No data	No data	Sedation, neutropenia, seizures, weight gain, metabolic syndrome.
Combination of medication + psychotherapy	2c, Hallucinations, delusions	No data	No data	No data	Same as monotherapies.

Note. Across all treatment studies for each type of child psychopathology, we used guidelines put forth by J. Cohen (1988): Strength of evidence: 1 = replicated clinical trial or large-body of single-subject studies; 2 = controlled clinical trial or replicated, single-subject study; 3 = comparison group but not clinical trial; 4 = no control group. Effect size: a = .81+, large; b = .51 to .80, medium; c = .21 to .50, small; d = .20 or less.
[a]Over 12 months. [b]See side effects and risk–benefit discussion.

Mueser & McGurk, 2004). Randomized double-blind studies are limited to haloperidol, clozapine, risperidone, and olanzapine. In the largest trial, 50 youths ages 8 to 19 with prominent psychotic symptoms were treated in an 8-week randomized double-blind parallel comparison of haloperidol, risperidone, and olanzapine. Treatment response was 53%, 74%, and 88%, respectively (Sikich, Hamer, Bashford, Sheitman, & Lieberman, 2004). Over 15 studies indicated the efficacy of clozapine in children and adolescents, but serious side effects occurred at a higher rate than in adults (for review, see Remschmidt, Hennighausen, Clement, Heiser, & Schultz, 2000). Ziprasidone may be beneficial in the treatment of psychosis (Meighen, Shelton, & McDougle, 2004). A large-scale, multicenter trial currently under way, Treatment of Early Onset Schizophrenia Spectrum Disorders, should shed more light on pharmacological intervention. In this four-site study, 165 youths ages 8 to 19 years are randomized to risperidone, olanzapine, or molindone for 8 weeks, with 2 or more weeks at a predetermined maximal dose. Those with a positive response continue under masked conditions for an additional 44 weeks. Findings have not been published but should provide information on safety and efficacy of three antipsychotic medications.

Strength of Evidence

Many studies include youths with psychotic symptoms but not necessarily schizophrenia spectrum disorders. Almost no studies include children under the age of 13. The number of studies is quite limited, and they deal only with acute outcomes, with the exception of one 2-year follow-up study of a comprehensive treatment program that used a historical control group that received an undocumented assortment of interventions.

Side Effects

All currently available medications carry the risk of serious side effects and must be monitored closely (McClellan et al., 2001). A serious yet common side effect of atypical antipsychotic medications is weight gain that can result in a series of general metabolic disorders, including Type 2 (non-insulin dependent) diabetes mellitus, lipid level changes, and transaminase elevation (Kowatch et al., 2005). The American Diabetes Association, in conjunction with the American Psychiatric Association, American Association of Clinical Endocrinologists, and North American Association for the Study of Obesity (2004), published a monitoring protocol for all individuals receiving atypical antipsychotic medications. There are anecdotal reports of cognitive side effects, including problems with word retrieval, working memory, and cognitive dulling (Kowatch et al., 2005). Neuroleptics may be associated with a shortened life span (Joukamaa et al., 2006). Other uncommon but problematic side effects associated with various medications that warrant careful monitoring include abnormal involuntary movements and prolactin elevation (antipsychotics), intracardiac conduction effects (ziprasidone), and hematological and neurological adverse side effects and neuroleptic malignant syndrome (clozapine).

COMBINED INTERVENTIONS

A combination of psychopharmacological and psychosocial treatment is recommended (Asarnow et al., 2004; McClellan et al., 2001), but the limited research in each respective area has not resulted in any determination of the relative efficacy of each treatment component in combination care. Promising initial findings were presented by McGorry et al. (2002). They provided combination low-dose risperidone and cognitive behavior therapy to 31 participants ages 14 to 28 (average age = 20 years) with subthreshold symptoms and compared their results with the results of 28 control participants who received needs-based intervention (supportive psychotherapy and case management). This combination treatment reduced the risk of early transition to psychosis, although the relative contributions of each intervention could not be determined.

Strength of Evidence

The level of evidence is currently rather limited as only a small, pilot, randomized, controlled trial has been reported in adolescents.

Limitations

No definitive controlled trials testing the effectiveness of combined interventions in youths with schizophrenia spectrum disorders have been conducted.

DIVERSITY

Given the small number of studies conducted on relatively small sample sizes, no meaningful comparisons have been made between treatment response for boys versus girls, or minority versus majority racial or ethnic groups. Further research examining treatment effects and outcomes by diversity variables is necessary.

RISK–BENEFIT ANALYSIS

The symptoms of schizophrenia spectrum disorders carry with them significant morbidity and mortality. Thus, adverse side effects associated with treatment must be weighed in light of the benefit the treatment provides. Given this, there is support for using pharmacological agents in well-monitored trials. There is no known risk of psychosocial interventions designed to aid the child and help the family cope with psychotic symptoms. Evidence suggests some psychosocial intervention can provide benefit.

FUTURE DIRECTIONS

Schizophrenia spectrum disorders are rare in childhood and uncommon in adolescents. Almost no empirical studies have examined psychosocial interventions and few have tested psychopharmacologic agents in children and adolescents. Psychosocial interventions that are psychoeducational, family-based, and cognitive–behavioral are suggested. Newer pharmacological agents hold promise for the future, although all carry the risk of serious side effects. Much more research is needed to develop optimal treatment guidelines for youths with schizophrenia-related disorders.

10

AUTISM SPECTRUM DISORDERS AND MENTAL RETARDATION

Autism spectrum disorders (ASDs) and *mental retardation* (MR) usually become apparent in the first 2 to 3 years of life. These problems are characterized by major deficits in cognitive abilities and communication, resulting in lifelong functional impairment. Most children with ASDs also have general cognitive deficits consistent with MR. According to the most recent estimates, the prevalence of autistic disorder is about 22 per 10,000, and ASDs (a broader category that includes autistic disorder) is about 60 per 10,000 (Chakrabarti & Fombonne, 2005; Yeargin-Allsopp et al., 2003). The prevalence of MR is estimated to range from 1% to 3% (Volkmar & Dykens, 2002).

PSYCHOSOCIAL INTERVENTIONS

Therapeutic interventions for children with ASDs and MR can be divided into two categories: (a) comprehensive treatment programs aimed at correcting the core deficits of ASDs and improving communication and interpersonal behavior and (b) ad hoc interventions to address behavioral problems like aggression, self-injury, stereotypes, and compulsions. Interventions are not curative and cannot fully correct the deficits of these disorders, but treatment can substantially improve functioning (Bryson, Rogers, & Fombonne, 2003; Koegel, Koegel, & Brookman, 2003; Lovaas & Smith, 2003; National Research Council, 2001).

A number of comprehensive treatment programs are in use for children with ASDs (Koegel & Koegel, 1995; Lovaas, 1987; National Research Council, 2001; Rogers & Lewis, 1989; Schopler & Mesibov, 1995). Although different in their theoretical foundation, these programs have common characteristics. Programs typically address multiple skill domains, involve 20 to 40 hours per week of direct instruction with parents on how to deliver the intervention, include structured teaching settings, emphasize early intervention (in preschool years), and last at least 2 years. Interventions include psychotherapy and educational elements.

Specific psychosocial interventions, mainly based on the principles of behavior therapy, are beneficial in decreasing symptoms (e.g., aggression, self-injury, compulsive behaviors) and improving functioning (Eikeseth, Smith, Jahr, & Eldevik, 2002; Kahng, Iwata, & Lewin, 2002; T. Smith, Groen, & Wynn, 2000). Table 10.1 provides a summary of treatment efficacy for autism spectrum disorders.

Strength of Evidence

Overall, the evidence for the efficacy of psychosocial interventions in ASDs and MR in decreasing symptoms and improving functioning is good but not as well documented through controlled clinical trials for conditions such as attention-deficit/hyperactivity disorder (ADHD). There are, in fact, only a few, relatively small, controlled clinical trials (Lovaas, 1987; T. Smith et al., 2000), and the evidence comes primarily from quasi-experimental designs and single-case studies. This damages any chance to compare effect sizes with a control condition. Nonetheless, researchers believe that these interventions can result in marked improvement. Myriad single-subject designs using operant techniques have demonstrated improvement in behaviors. Future research needs to incorporate these techniques into controlled clinical trials. Psychosocial interventions constitute the mainstay of treatment for children with ASDs, but larger and more representative controlled studies to test their efficacy are needed (Lord et al., 2005).

Limitations

Even though these interventions can lead to major improvements, especially in the domains of communication and general behavior, complete remediation of the core deficits of autism has not been and is unlikely to be achieved. Moreover, comprehensive treatments are expensive and require

TABLE 10.1
Treatment Efficacy for Autism Spectrum Disorders (ASDs) and Mental Retardation

	Acute		Long term[a]		
Treatment	Strength of evidence and effect size, Primary symptoms	Strength of evidence and effect size, Functional outcomes	Strength of evidence and effect size, Primary symptoms	Strength of evidence and effect size, Functional outcomes	Side effects[b]
Psychosocial	1a, Self-injurious behavior, severe tantrum, stereotypies, language and communication social skills	1a, Improve functioning in interpersonal, academic, and other adaptive behaviors	3c, Self-injurious behavior, severe tantrum, stereotypies, language and communication social skills	3c, Improve functioning in interpersonal, academic, and other adaptive behaviors	Usually well tolerated but limited data.
Medication					
Methylphenidate	1c, Inattention, hyperactivity, impulsiveness	4d	No data	No data	More adverse side effects (irritability, social withdrawal, affective blunting, insomnia) than with non-ASD.
Risperidone	1a, Self-injurious behavior, severe tantrum, stereotypies	1a, General functioning by decreasing aggression	No data	No data	Neurological adverse events, weight gain, sedation, increased risk for diabetes.
Clomipramine	2c, perseverative behavior	No data	No data	No data	Sedation
Fluoxetine	2c, perseverative behavior	No data	No data	No data	Irritability
Combination	No data	No data	No data	No data	No data

Note. Across all treatment studies for each type of child psychopathology, we used guidelines put forth by J. Cohen (1988): Strength of evidence: 1 = replicated clinical trial or large-body, single-subject study; 2 = controlled clinical trial or replicated, single-subject study; 3 = comparison group but not clinical trial; 4 = no control group. Effect size: a = .81+, large; b = .51 to .80, medium; c = .21 to .50, small; d = .20 or less.
[a]Over 12 months. [b]See side effects and risk–benefit discussion.

highly trained staff and substantial commitment from the family. Nonetheless, the cost of these therapies may still far outweigh the adverse side effects of pharmacological treatments and so deserve careful attention.

PHARMACOLOGICAL INTERVENTIONS

Rather than correct the core deficits of the disorder, pharmacotherapy is an ancillary intervention to control ASD behaviors such as aggression, self-injury, tantrums, impulsiveness, and stereotypic-compulsive behavior. These behaviors are common among children with ASDs and MR and cause substantial impairment. Attempts to develop pharmacological interventions to correct the core communication deficits of ASDs and MR have not been successful, as shown in the examples of fenfluramine, naltrexone, and secretin (Campbell et al., 1988; Sandler et al., 1999; Sturmey, 2005). Ongoing research on the pathogenesis of autism and related disorders may indicate more promise for future drug development.

Despite their ancillary role, psychotropic medications are commonly used in the treatment of children with ASDs and MR. In fact, epidemiological community surveys indicate that 33% to 47% of children with ASDs receive at least one psychotropic medication during a 1-year period (Aman, Lam, & Collier-Crespin, 2003; Aman, Lam, & Van Bourgondien, 2005; Witwer & Lecavalier, 2005). The most commonly used psychotropic medications in ASDs are antidepressants, antipsychotics, stimulants, and the alpha agonist clonidine. Also used are mood stabilizers, such as lithium and divalproex sodium. The strength of the evidence for the efficacy of these medications is variable, ranging from placebo-controlled clinical trials to open-label case reports.

Stimulants are used to control symptoms of hyperactivity, impulsiveness, and inattention commonly encountered in children with ASDs and MR, even though the *Diagnostic and Statistical Manual of Mental Disorders* (4th ed., text rev.; American Psychiatric Association, 2000) nosological perspective does not permit a formal diagnosis of ADHD in the context of a pervasive developmental disorder. A recently completed, publicly funded, multisite, controlled clinical trial provided evidence that methylphenidate was efficacious in relieving ADHD symptoms in children with ASDs, but its efficacy and tolerability were more variable than in children with ADHD but no developmental disorder (Research Units on Pediatric Psychopharmacology [RUPP] Autism Network, 2005a). Approximately 50% of children with ASDs had a positive response to methylphenidate, and about 18% had adverse side effects, some of which were highly disruptive but short-lived.

A 4-week, placebo-controlled within-subject study compared methylphenidate, administered at different doses, with placebo. Of the 72 children who entered the study, 18% interrupted treatment because of adverse side effects, and 48% showed clinically significant improvement. These rates contrast with a discontinuation rate caused by adverse side effects of less than 5% and an improvement rate of more than 70% in hyperactive children without pervasive developmental disorders (Greenhill et al., 2001).

Antipsychotic medications, antidopaminergic agents marketed for the treatment of psychosis in adults, are commonly used off-label to treat aggression and severe tantrums in children. Typical antipsychotics have been used for decades to control behavioral problems in children with MR and ASDs. In particular, placebo-controlled studies document the efficacy of haloperidol in autism (L. T. Anderson et al., 1989).

In more recent years, atypical antipsychotics, such as risperidone, have gradually replaced the typical antipsychotic medications. Evidence from a multisite, controlled, publicly funded clinical trial shows that risperidone is efficacious in decreasing severe behavioral disturbances in 5- to 17-year-old children with autism (RUPP Autism Network, 2002, 2005b). About two thirds of children treated with risperidone improved, compared with 12% on placebo at the end of the 8-week trial. Shea et al. (2004) essentially replicated these findings in a group of children with autism, pervasive developmental disorder not otherwise specified, or Asperger's syndrome, none of whom were selected for extremely disruptive behavior.

The beneficial effect seen by the RUPP Autism Network (2002) was sustained through the 6 months of treatment, but the behavioral problems usually recurred when the medication was discontinued. This long-term effect while on medication was recently replicated by an independent group of researchers (Troost et al., 2005). The research tends to show that risperidone is efficacious but noncurative. Also, it is associated with weight gain, which can make long-term treatment problematic. The efficacy of other antipsychotics has been less well investigated and is currently limited to uncontrolled studies.

Selective serotonin reuptake inhibitors (SSRIs), such as clomipramine, fluoxetine, and fluvoxamine, have been used in the treatment of compulsive repetitive behaviors. We have limited evidence from small controlled trials that clomipramine and fluoxetine are efficacious for managing perseverative behaviors (compulsions, stereotypes, and self-injury) in children with autism (Gordon, State, Nelson, Hamburger, & Rapoport, 1993; Hollander et al., 2005). Fluoxetine had a more favorable tolerability profile than clomipramine, and there is some uncertainty whether children and adolescents respond as well as adults (Aman, Arnold, & Armstrong, 1999). Further controlled investigations are ongoing on the efficacy of SSRIs in reducing repetitive behaviors and improving general functioning of children with ASDs.

Clonidine and the pharmacologically related guanfacine are alpha agonists that are marketed for the treatment of hypertension in adults but are also used off-label to treat hyperactivity in children. These drugs are often used in children with ASDs in an attempt to control hyperactivity, aggression, and severe tantrums. At this time, their efficacy is supported only by open-label, uncontrolled reports (Posey & McDougle, 2001).

Mood stabilizers like lithium and divalproate are also used in children with ASDs and MR for the control of explosive aggression and severe tantrums. These medications are effective treatments for adults with bipolar disorders, but despite their use in children with ASDs and MR, conclusive evidence for their efficacy in youths does not exist. No randomized controlled trials in children and adolescents with ASDs or MR are available to support efficacy. A few small trials in adults provide preliminary support for their efficacy.

Strength of Evidence

Randomized controlled studies strongly support the efficacy of antipsychotics and stimulants in decreasing symptoms of disruptive behavior in children (ages 5 and older) and adolescents. The effect of antipsychotics is large (i.e., Cohen's effect size above .8) and that of stimulants is more modest (effect sizes between .2 and .5). Less clear is the impact of these agents on functioning. In a randomized trial, treatment with risperidone resulted in improvement in the restricted and repetitive patterns of behavior but did not change the deficits in communication and social interactions that are typical of autism (McDougle et al., 2005).

Side Effects

The medications used in the management of children with ASDs or MR have distinctive side effects that are related to the pharmacological activities of these agents. In some cases, there is evidence that the risk–benefit ratio of these medications is less favorable for children with ASDs than for children without ASDs. For instance, adverse side effects, primarily agitation, irritability, and insomnia, led to discontinuation of methylphenidate in 18% of children with ASDs ages 5 to 14 years (RUPP Autism Network, 2005a). This discontinuation rate is substantially higher than that reported in children who are diagnosed with ADHD (less than 2%).

In general, children with ASDs and MR can be considered at increased risk for drug-induced side effects because their brains are likely to be more sensitive to pharmacological intervention. These children contend with underlying developmental disturbance, and their deficits in communication can impair or delay recognition of drug toxicities. Two types of adverse side effects are noteworthy for antipsychotics, which have the best evidence for efficacy. These are neurological toxicities for typical antipsychotics (i.e., dystonias, dyskinesias, tremor, Parkinsonism, and akathisia) and weight gain for commonly used atypical antipsychotics such as risperidone and olanzapine.

The latter drugs may also increase the risk for metabolic disturbances like diabetes and hyperlipidemia (American Diabetes Association et al., 2004).

COMBINED INTERVENTIONS

Psychosocial and psychopharmacological interventions are often used conjunctively, but little is currently known about the interactions between these two treatment modalities. For instance, it is not known whether medications enhance the efficacy of psychosocial treatment or whether psychosocial treatment allows medication to be discontinued eventually without recurrence of symptoms.

DIVERSITY

Data do not currently exist on the effect of treatment by subject subgroups. In general, sample sizes have been too small to be able to detect subgroup differences. Further research with larger sample sizes examining treatment effects and outcomes by diversity variables is necessary.

RISK–BENEFIT ANALYSIS

The balance between risk and benefit clearly favors psychosocial interventions and is also generally favorable for selected medications, such as antipsychotics and stimulants, when used in the short term (2–6 months). Data on longer term use are lacking. Psychopharmacological interventions are often less favorable for children with ASDs or MR than for nondevelopmentally impaired peers. For instance, stimulants and SSRIs are generally less well tolerated by children with ASDs as compared with peers with ADHD or anxiety disorders.

A corpus of research exists in the field of ASDs and MR related to behavior therapy. Not many controlled clinical trials compare behavior therapy with no treatment, but studies in the field of applied behavior analysis (ABA) that have used ABA designs have yielded impressive data on the efficacy of operant techniques. This is especially true when specific symptoms that are associated with these disorders are targeted. We refer interested readers to Baumeister and Baumeister (1995), Harris (1995), and Kobe and Mulick (1995).

The determination of risk–benefit for psychotropic use in children with ASDs and MR must be made at the level of the individual child and must take certain factors into consideration. These include the medication side-effect profile, severity of the symptoms, level of dysfunction, response to alternative and nonpharmacological treatment, and current medical condition (e.g., risperidone may not be appropriate for an obese child).

FUTURE DIRECTIONS

Further research is suggested on the effectiveness of existing comprehensive interventions, specifically the extent of the improvement these interventions can provide, the identification of subgroups of children most likely to benefit from them, the relationship between the intensity of treatment and treatment outcome, and the overall cost–benefit analyses (Lord et al., 2005). In addition, it is necessary to apply neuroscience findings to the development of psychosocial, educational, and pharmacological treatments to address the core symptoms of ASDs and MR in an evidence-based and effective way.

11

ANOREXIA NERVOSA AND BULIMIA NERVOSA

Anorexia nervosa may arise in children as young as 8 years of age; *bulimia nervosa* rarely appears before the age of 12 (Gowers & Bryant-Waugh, 2004). More common than full-blown eating disorders are clinically significant symptoms that may include a highly focused preoccupation with food, weight, or shape and some sort of disordered eating. The prevalence of anorexia nervosa in girls seems to be between .3% and 1%, peaking during the ages of 15 to 19, with a girl-to-boy ratio of about 11:1 (W. G. Johnson, Tsoh, & Varnado, 1996; Van Hoeken, Seidell, & Hoek, 2003). The prevalence of bulimia nervosa seems to be 1% to 3%, with a girl-to-boy ratio of about 30:1 (Gowers & Bryant-Waugh, 2004; W. G. Johnson et al., 1996).

Depression is commonly associated with eating disorders. Approximately 45% of individuals with anorexia nervosa and up to 88% of those with bulimia nervosa have a lifetime history of mood disorder (Pike & Striegel-Moore, 1997). Depressive symptoms do not appear to influence outcome (Gowers & Bryant-Waugh, 2004). However, obsessive–compulsive disorder (OCD) and residual OCD symptoms are associated with poorer outcome. Comorbid anxiety disorders seem to be at least as common as depression, with two thirds of all individuals diagnosed as having an eating disorder also meeting criteria for one or more lifetime anxiety disorders, most commonly OCD or social phobia (Kaye et al., 2004).

PSYCHOSOCIAL INTERVENTIONS

The evidence for treatment efficacy of anorexia nervosa across all age groups is weak, with very few randomized controlled trials (Gowers & Bryant-Waugh, 2004; Treasure & Schmidt, 2003). Only a few, small controlled studies have been reported in adolescents with anorexia nervosa. Russell, Szmukler, Dare, and Eisler (1987) compared 13 sessions of family therapy with individual therapy in 21 youths (mean age = 17 years). Improvement rate was 90% with family therapy versus 18% with individual therapy. Another study with 37 youths (mean age = 14 years) found an improvement rate of 81% with family therapy versus 66% with individual therapy (Robin et al., 1999). A study with 40 youths (mean age = 15 years) compared whole family therapy with separate family therapy, with no difference found in response rate between the two (Eisler et al., 2000).

On the basis of existing, somewhat limited evidence, it appears that behavioral family therapy may be considered a reasonable first-line approach to anorexia nervosa in adolescence. In the few extant controlled studies, clinicians must extrapolate from data that include adults to design evidence-based treatments for children. A review by Treasure and Schmidt (2003) showed limited evidence from one randomized controlled trial that focal therapy, cognitive-analytic therapy, and family therapy were more effective than treatment-as-usual in adults. Another small randomized controlled trial showed outpatient treatment was as effective as inpatient treatment in adolescents and adults who did not need emergency medical treatment (Treasure & Schmidt, 2003). No differences were found between various psychotherapies or between psychotherapy and dietary advice in another 10 randomized controlled trials (Treasure & Schmidt, 2003). In McIntosh et al. (2005), a randomized controlled trial with a mostly adult sample that included girls with anorexia nervosa as young as 17 years old found that nonspecific supportive clinical management was superior to either cognitive behavior therapy (CBT) or interpersonal therapy (IPT).

Several systematic reviews of bulimia nervosa treatments are available, but no randomized controlled trials involving adolescents have been published (Gowers & Bryant-Waugh, 2004). These reviews have found that CBT is an effective intervention for the purging and eating behaviors of bulimia nervosa and associated symptoms such as depression. CBT usually involves psychoeducation, self-monitoring, application of behavioral strategies to establish more regular eating habits (e.g., self-reward for three meals plus two snacks at regular times of the day), elimination of rigid dieting, and strategies to decrease bingeing and purging. Treatment may include stimulus control strategies to help the person avoid or change situations that typically trigger a binge or purge. Treatment may also involve addressing cognitive distortions (e.g., certain foods are good or bad) and using exposure techniques for avoided food or anxiety-evoking situations. IPT, though also beneficial, has resulted in more modest effects. Table 11.1 provides a summary of treatment efficacy for anorexia and bulimia nervosa.

Strength of Evidence

The evidence for psychosocial interventions for anorexia nervosa is weak, as it is based primarily on case series or other uncontrolled reports. There are only a few randomized controlled trials with children and few outcome studies of any kind in individuals with anorexia nervosa. The evidence for psychosocial interventions in bulimia nervosa is much stronger, although there are no studies with children specifically, forcing clinicians to extrapolate from adult data. The effects sizes of psychosocial interventions in the acute treatment of bulimia nervosa are moderate. There are not enough data to make conclusions about long-term follow-up.

Limitations

In some cases, because of concerns about physical safety, patients may need to be hospitalized until treatment has been determined to be efficacious and there are no longer dangers to individual health and well-being. Also, it is fairly common for treated patients to continue to experience persistent subthreshold symptoms (e.g., Jager, Liedtke, Lamprecht, & Freyberger, 2004). Unfortunately, psychosocial interventions may be a limited resource in some communities.

PHARMACOLOGICAL INTERVENTIONS

Ten studies of controlled drug trials, usually tricyclic antidepressants (TCAs) or selective serotonin reuptake inhibitors (SSRIs), with individuals with anorexia nervosa failed to document efficacy in terms of physical and psychological outcome (Treasure & Schmidt, 2003). Fluoxetine reduced the risk of relapse after weight restoration in adults with anorexia nervosa (Kaye et al., 2001). However, an observational, 2-year longitudinal follow-up of adults with anorexia nervosa did not show any benefit of antidepressant treatment for relapse (Strober, Freeman, DeAntonio, Lampert, & Diamond, 1997).

In bulimia nervosa and binge eating disorder, W. G. Johnson et al. (1996) showed that antidepressants reduced bingeing and purging, although this result seems independent of any antidepressant effect. Other reviews of antidepressant trials (Bacaltchuk, Hay, & Mari, 2000; Whittal, Agras, & Gould,

TABLE 11.1
Treatment Efficacy for Anorexia Nervosa and Bulimia Nervosa

	Acute		Long term[a]		
Treatment	Strength of evidence and effect size, Primary symptoms	Strength of evidence and effect size, Functional outcomes	Strength of evidence and effect size, Primary symptoms	Strength of evidence and effect size, Functional outcomes	Side effects[b]
Psychosocial	2c, Anorexia nervosa	2c	No data	No data	No data
	2b, Bulimia nervosa	2b	2b	No data	No data
Medication	4d, Anorexia nervosa	4d	No data	No data	No data
	2b, Bulimia nervosa	2b	2d	No data	No data
Combination	No data, Anorexia nervosa	No data	No data	No data	No data
	2b, Bulimia nervosa	2b	No data	No data	No data

Note. Across all treatment studies for each type of child psychopathology, we used guidelines put forth by J. Cohen (1988): Strength of evidence: 1 = replicated clinical trial or large-body, single-subject study; 2 = controlled clinical trial or replicated, single-subject study; 3 = comparison group but not clinical trial; 4 = no control group. Effect size: a = .81+, large; b = .51 to .80, medium; c = .21 to .50, small; d = .20 or less.
[a]Over 12 months. [b]See side effects and risk–benefit discussion.

1999) found short-term improvements in bulimic symptoms and a small improvement in depressive symptoms. TCAs, SSRIs, and monoamine oxidase inhibitors had comparable efficacy and tolerability (Bacaltchuk et al., 2000). Atypical antipsychotics, especially olanzapine, have been tried in open-label, nonrandomized single-case studies, some of which were with adolescents (Barbarich et al., 2004; Mehler et al., 2001). Results from these studies suggest a possible benefit of olanzapine in increasing weight and decreasing weight obsession. CBT also reduced bingeing and purging, and direct comparisons with medication alone favored CBT, particularly when longer term follow-up is considered (W. G. Johnson et al., 1996).

Strength of Evidence

The evidence for psychopharmacological interventions for anorexia nervosa is very weak to nonexistent. There are no randomized controlled trials targeting children and few outcome studies of any kind to use for guidance in treating patients with anorexia. The evidence for psychopharmacological interventions in bulimia nervosa is much stronger, although there are no studies with children specifically. The effect sizes for psychopharmacological interventions in the acute treatment of bulimia nervosa are moderate. There are not enough data to make conclusions about longer term follow-up.

Side Effects

The side effects of antidepressants are delineated in the chapter on depressive disorders (chap. 7). Side effects in patients with eating disorders are not expected to be demonstrably different from those in patients with depression. The black box warnings about increased risk of suicidality apply to the use of all antidepressants in children, regardless of the problem being treated. On the basis of adult studies (Lieberman et al., 2005), up to 70% of patients who take atypical antipsychotics (e.g., olanzapine) experience moderate to severe side effects. These include insomnia (16%), sleepiness (30%), urinary hesitancy, dry mouth, constipation (24%), sexual problems (27%), menstrual irregularities (36%), and orthostatic faintness (9%). Up to 30% of patients taking olanzapine experienced a weight gain of more than 7%, raising risk for diabetes and other weight-related problems (Lieberman et al., 2005).

COMBINED INTERVENTIONS

No studies have systematically evaluated the efficacy of combining psychosocial and pharmacological interventions for anorexia nervosa. Bacaltchuk et al. (2000) found evidence for the superiority of combining psychotherapy and antidepressants over antidepressants alone for bulimia nervosa in terms of remission rate and mood symptoms but not in reducing binge frequency. Given the preponderance of the evidence, CBT would appear to be the treatment of first choice for bulimia nervosa in children and adolescents, typically resulting in a recovery rate of 40% to 50% (D. A. Anderson & Maloney, 2001) compared with a recovery rate of only about 19% with antidepressants alone (Bacaltchuk et al., 2000).

DIVERSITY

Minimal data exist on the role of ethnicity or racial background for children and adolescents with eating disorders. Some data show that ethnic minority women who seek treatment for anorexia nervosa have lower admission weights than White women, suggesting that anorexia nervosa may go undetected or untreated longer in ethnic minority women (Pike & Striegel-Moore, 1997). Often considered a disorder of White, affluent girls from Western cultures, bulimia nervosa appears to be increasing among non-White groups, including African Americans and women in developing non-Western cultures (Pike & Striegel-Moore, 1997).

Subgroups of youths, such as gymnasts, models, and dancers, may be more at risk for developing bulimia nervosa because of cultural pressure to conform to a certain body image and the stringent physical requirements of the roles (Pike & Striegel-Moore, 1997). Better prognosis in bulimia nervosa has been associated with shorter duration of the disorder, less severe symptoms, higher social class, younger onset, family history of alcoholism, high self-esteem, and lower perfectionism (Gowers & Bryant-Waugh, 2004). Efforts should be made to include boys in treatment outcome studies of eating disorders. Further research examining treatment effects and outcomes by diversity variables is necessary.

RISK–BENEFIT ANALYSIS

There are not many controlled studies in the treatment of anorexia nervosa, perhaps because of the practical challenges of conducting such research. This necessitates that clinicians rely on expert opinion. On the basis of reviews of the treatment outcome literature, to achieve recovery in bulimia nervosa compared with placebo, the number needed to benefit one additional child (NNTB) for CBT seems to be about 3; for antidepressants, about 9. Not enough data are available to calculate the number needed to treat to cause harm in one additional child (NNTH) for combination treatment. Compared with placebo, the NNTH for antidepressants in terms of treatment discontinuation due to an adverse effect seems to be about 19 (Bacaltchuk et al., 2000). There are no comparable data to allow an NNTH calculation for psychosocial treatment, although adverse medical effects are expected to be lower than those for antidepressant medications.

FUTURE DIRECTIONS

Future research needs to determine precisely the effectiveness of specific forms of family therapy in anorexia nervosa and the value of SSRI medication in decreasing risk for recurrence in patients who have reached remission. Promising results of guided self-help interventions for bulimia nervosa, usually those based on CBT, should be pursued with haste (Hay, Bacaltchuk, & Stefano, 2004). Research should also examine ethnic and cultural influences on eating disorders in general and on response to treatment in particular. Randomized controlled trials for the treatment of anorexia nervosa are especially needed to examine the relative efficacy of medication versus psychosocial interventions alone and then in combination. In September 2005, the National Institute of Mental Health funded a cooperative agreement to conduct a multisite clinical trial of a specific form of family behavioral therapy (the Maudsley approach) in more than 200 adolescents with anorexia nervosa. The expected duration of this study is 5 years.

12

ELIMINATION DISORDERS

Elimination disorders include nocturnal enuresis and encopresis. *Nocturnal enuresis* is defined as repeated urination into bed or clothes, which occurs at least twice per week for at least 3 consecutive months, in a child who is at least 5 years of age and where the condition is not due to either a drug side effect or medical condition (American Psychiatric Association, 2000). Nocturnal enuresis is especially common during early childhood years. Approximately 15% to 20% of 5-year-olds and 7% to 15% of 7-year-olds are enuretic at least once per month. Ondersma and Walker (1998) found that about 7% of 7-year-old boys and 3% of 7-year-old girls were enuretic weekly. In addition, 3% of children with enuresis remain incontinent well into adulthood (Mellon & Houts, 1998). *Diurnal enuresis* is much less frequent than nocturnal enuresis, with nocturnal enuresis being more common among girls and occurring in approximately 1% of 6- to 12-year-olds.

Encopresis is defecation in inappropriate places over a given time occurring at least once per month for at least 3 months (American Psychiatric Association, 2000). The child must be at least 4 years of age and the behavior must not be exclusively due to the side effects of medications or physical problems other than constipation. The diagnosis of encopresis also requires a determination of whether the soiling is due to constipation. Among 5-year-olds, the American Psychiatric Association (2000) estimated 1% have encopresis, and the disorder is 5 to 6 times more prevalent among boys. Referrals for encopresis account for approximately 3% of youths, and 5% of these referrals are to psychiatric clinics (Franklin & Johnson, 2003). Frequency of encopresis decreases with age, with a spontaneous remission rate of about 28% per year (Franklin & Johnson, 2003).

PSYCHOSOCIAL INTERVENTIONS

Given the potential for some type of organic etiology for enuresis and encopresis, a practitioner should partner with a pediatrician in assessing and managing enuresis and encopresis. Operant techniques have been successful in the management of enuresis and encopresis. A number of reviews and numerous well-controlled clinical trials have clearly documented the importance and efficacy of the urine alarm as an important treatment for enuresis, in combination with dry-bed training, which is a basic operant approach to the management of enuresis (for a review, see Mellon & McGrath, 2000). Full-spectrum home training is one multicomponent treatment approach that includes the urine alarm and other components, including retention and control training with monetary rewards, cleanliness training, self-monitoring of wet and dry nights, and a graduated overlearning procedure. These approaches are manualized, and an advantage of this multicomponent treatment approach over the urine alarm treatment alone is the inclusion of components designed to reduce relapse after successful therapy (for a review, see Mellon & McGrath, 2000). Approaches focusing on enhancing compliance that include a cognitive approach (e.g., hypnotic interventions) clearly warrant further investigation.

Well-established interventions for encopresis have not been documented, although researchers have identified several probable efficacious therapies and three promising interventions. Two specific medical interventions (one with a fiber recommendation and one without; Loening-Baucke, 1989) with positive reinforcement are likely efficacious treatments for encopresis (Waid, Chandra, Gabel, & Chapin, 1987). Biofeedback in combination with medical interventions has shown promise in the management of constipation with abnormal defecation (Cox, Sutphen, Borowitz, Kovatchev, & Ling, 1998). Other promising interventions for encopresis include correction of paradoxical contraction, positive reinforcement, dietary education, goal setting, and skills building focused on relaxation during defecation. Table 12.1 provides a summary of treatment efficacy for elimination disorders.

Strength of Evidence

The basic urine alarm alone is considered to be necessary in the treatment of enuresis and, in combination with the dry-bed training, is an effec-

TABLE 12.1
Treatment Efficacy for Elimination Disorders

Treatment	Strength of evidence and effect size, Primary symptoms	Strength of evidence and effect size, Functional outcomes	Side effects[a]
Psychosocial			
Urine alarm	Enuresis	1a	None reported
Dry-bed training	No data	1a	None reported
Full-spectrum home training	Encopresis	1b	None reported
Positive reinforcement	Encopresis	2b	None reported
Biofeedback	2b	No data	None reported
Correction of paradoxical contraction	3c	No data	None reported
Dietary education	4c	No data	None reported
Goal setting	4c	No data	None reported
Skill building	4c	No data	None reported
Medication			
Imipramine	Enuresis	2b	Cardiac conduction disturbances, orthostatic hypotension.
DDAVP	Enuresis	2b	None reported
Combination			
Urine alarm with DDAVP	4a, Enuresis	No data	None reported

Note. Across all treatment studies for each type of child psychopathology, we used guidelines put forth by J. Cohen (1988): Strength of evidence: 1 = replicated clinical trial or large-body, single-subject study; 2 = controlled clinical trial or replicated, single-subject study; 3 = comparison group but not clinical trial; 4 = no control group. Effect size: a = .81+, large; b = .51 to .80, medium; c = .21 to .50, small; d = .20 or less. DDAVP = a synthetic vasopressin (also known as desmopressin).
[a]See side effects and risk–benefit discussion.

tive treatment (Mellon & McGrath, 2000). Also, full-spectrum home training improves outcome for children with enuresis but is classified only as probably efficacious because other studies have not replicated the data from the full-spectrum home training behavioral intervention. Other approaches that focus on improving compliance with treatment or that incorporate a cognitive focus warrant investigation, although no information is available as to their strength of evidence.

By contrast to the enuresis literature, in the management of constipation and encopresis, no well-established investigations are available in the extant literature. Specifically, medical interventions that include positive reinforcement and interventions that include biofeedback have been considered probably efficacious (McGrath, Mellon, & Murphy, 2000).

The behavioral approaches in the management of enuresis and encopresis are the most successful compared with other therapies, including pharmacotherapy, in the immediate management of symptoms and ensuring durability once therapy has ceased.

Limitations

The efficacy of the urine alarm in the management of nocturnal enuresis is well documented in a number of compelling literature reviews (Doleys, 1977; Houts, Berman, & Abramson, 1994; S. B. Johnson, 1980; Mellon & McGrath, 2000; Moffatt, 1997). However, patient characteristics predicting best treatment outcome for the alarm remain unclear. Further, it is unclear whether other components of treatment add to the effectiveness of the urine alarm. The interaction of enuresis and the frequently occurring comorbid physical conditions, including delays in central nervous system development, of children with enuresis in the context of learning theory remains unknown (Mellon & McGrath, 2000).

Limitations of psychosocial interventions for encopresis include the failure of clinical trials to delineate specific symptoms (e.g., incontinence, constipation, abnormal defecation) that are especially responsive to specific behavioral interventions. In addition, the role of adherence on the part of families is unclear, which is crucial to success or failure in treatment outcome. Given that disease management has been associated with family functioning, the role of the family in predicting treatment outcome is of utmost importance. Insufficient information is available on severity and duration of encopresis and how this is influenced by behavioral approaches.

PHARMACOLOGICAL INTERVENTIONS

There are no available pharmacotherapies that specifically target encopresis with the exception of agents that manage constipation. One of the first pharmacotherapies successfully used for the pharmacological management of enuresis was imipramine. Nonetheless, because of serious side effects, including cardiac toxicity and other known toxicities associated with tricyclic antidepressants, synthetic vasopressin (DDAVP, also known as desmopressin) soon replaced imipramine as the pharmacotherapy of choice for the management of enuresis. Because the synthesis of this medication was especially costly in oral tablet form (a great deal of the compound would be needed for the purpose of achieving adequate blood levels), a nasal spray was soon developed. Even though DDAVP is efficacious in many cases in the management of enuresis, once the medication is withdrawn, the child almost always reverts to wetting (Moffatt, Harlos, Kirshen, & Burd, 1993). Thus, durability is clearly in the short term with no generalization or expectation of durability in the long term.

There are no available studies examining the combination of either imipramine or DDAVP, the basic two pharmacotherapies demonstrated to be efficacious in the management of enuresis, in combination with operant approaches. Although medical interventions designed to reduce constipation are frequently used simultaneously with behavioral approaches and biofeedback to manage encopresis, no specific pharmacological agent has been studied with behavioral approaches that targeted encopresis. For this reason, behavior therapy is necessary even if it is used only adjunctively to pharmacotherapy.

Strength of Evidence

The strength of evidence on the use of pharmacotherapy in the short-term management of enuresis is that pharmacotherapy is an effective treatment only for enuresis; there are no known psychotropic medications for encopresis.

Side Effects

Prior to the U.S. Food and Drug Administration's approval of DDAVP for use for enuresis in children and adolescents, imipramine (a tricyclic antidepressant; Tofranil) was the most frequently used medication for bed-wetting. Because of sudden deaths involving cardiac complications in children being treated with imipramine (Varley & McClellan, 1997), imipramine is no longer considered a satisfactory or a viable treatment for the management of enuresis in children and adolescents. Desmopressin, which results in significant reductions in urine output, does have some adverse side effects that include transient headaches and nausea.

Limitations in the pharmacotherapy of enuresis include the high cost of treatment, the fact that the pharmacotherapies rarely stop bedwetting, and that upon cessation of pharmacotherapy, the child experiences complete relapse (Moffatt et al., 1993). Relapse is almost always demoralizing.

COMBINED INTERVENTIONS

As Mellon and McGrath (2000) observed, the combination of the urine alarm with DDAVP offers significant promise and may push the already high success rates of conditioning approaches to nearly 100%. In support of this conclusion, Woo and Park (2004) examined the efficacy of a urine alarm for the management of enuresis as a second-line therapeutic approach for children who failed to respond to pharmacotherapy. After using the urine alarm with children who had failed to improve with a trial of pharmacotherapy, over 90% of partial responders became full responders. These findings support the high success rates of behavioral treatments for the management of enuresis. No conclusions can be made with regard to strength of evidence of combined psychosocial and psychopharmacological treatments because not enough research is available.

DIVERSITY

With the exception of the research focused on the difference in the prevalence of enuresis and encopresis among boys and girls (Franklin & Johnson, 2003; Ondersma & Walker, 1998), no studies have focused specifically on pharmacotherapies or nonpharmacological therapies as they are associated with gender, ethnicity, or race. Treatment response also has not been studied as a function of gender, race, or ethnicity. Further research examining treatment effects and outcomes by diversity variables is necessary.

RISK–BENEFIT ANALYSIS

Given the strength of evidence associated with behavioral approaches for the management of enuresis and the limited side effects of these therapies documented in the extant literature, behavioral approaches are concluded to be of high benefit and of little risk in the management of enuresis and encopresis in youths. In the short and long term, a number of risks have been associated with imipramine that could result in problems with cardiac conduction, including death. Because of concerns about cardiac toxicity associated with imipramine, DDAVP has replaced imipramine as a pharmacotherapy for enuresis and is efficacious in the short term, although there is limited investigation about the safety of this agent in either the short or the long term. Thus, the benefit of behavior therapy appears to be especially high for both enuresis and encopresis, and the benefit of pharmacotherapy for enuresis is not especially high. No psychopharmacotherapy has been demonstrated to be efficacious in the management of encopresis.

FUTURE DIRECTIONS

It is clear that a future direction for treatment research in the area of elimination disorders will include studies that can examine the individual and combined treatments of medical interventions (e.g., pharmacotherapy for enuresis, laxatives, high fiber diets for encopresis) and psychosocial treatments for the management of enuresis and encopresis. It will be important to conduct clinical trials that have an adequate number of participants across age groups, which will allow for a comparison of both medical treatments employed alone, psychosocial treatments employed alone, as well as the combination of both psychosocial and medical therapies. Furthermore, the role of the family in assuring adherence to treatment will be necessary for systematic examination.

13

FUTURE DIRECTIONS AND IMPLICATIONS

Empirical evidence and clinical experience support the therapeutic benefit of psychosocial and pharmacological interventions for the treatment of children and adolescents with mental disorders. Researchers have recently advanced the knowledge of treatment for the most common childhood disorders, providing better guidance to clinicians and improving practitioners' ability to make better and more informed treatment decisions. For many interventions, the short-term efficacy is fairly well demonstrated. In contrast, evidence supporting the acute effect of treatment on daily life and the long-term effect on symptoms and outcomes is less well documented. In particular, safety remains a concern for a number of psychopharmacological interventions.

MAJOR UNANSWERED QUESTIONS

An important question is which treatment to use first. The answer is critical in determining, for example, how many children need and receive a particular intervention when two exist. Moreover, given that many parents and caregivers have preferences about treatments for their children, the sequences in which treatments are initiated are of paramount importance to families.

Algorithms recommending particular treatment sequences abound (American Academy of Child & Adolescent Psychiatry, 2002; American Academy of Pediatrics, 2001b). The American Academy of Child & Adolescent Psychiatry guideline on treatment of bipolar disorder recommends medication and psychosocial interventions be used simultaneously. The American Academy of Pediatrics guideline for attention-deficit/hyperactivity disorder (ADHD) recommends that treatment for ADHD should involve medication, behavior therapy, or their combination, without a sequence specified. However, none of these algorithms for treatment sequencing are evidence-based—a result of the fact that to our knowledge there are no published studies in which different sequences or simultaneous implementations of multiple modalities have been systematically compared. Existing recommendations for treatment sequencing are thus based only on expert consensus.

In the absence of empirical evidence, we believe that the choice and order of treatments (including absence of treatment) should be in general guided by the balance between anticipated benefit and possible harm. The safest treatments with demonstrated efficacy should be considered first before other treatments with less favorable profiles are considered. For most of the disorders reviewed in this book, psychosocial treatments are solidly grounded in empirical support as stand-alone treatments. Moreover, the preponderance of evidence indicates that psychosocial treatments are safer than psychoactive medications. Thus, it is our recommendation that in most cases psychosocial interventions be considered first.

The acute and long-term safety and efficacy data available for each disorder will be central to this decision. Cultural and individual differences must be included in all decision making on safety and efficacy data, and families might weigh them differently. It is ultimately the families' choice about which treatments to use and in which order. A clinician's role is to provide every family with the best and most recent evidence about short- and long-term risks and benefits of treatments. As the evidence continues to grow, it is hoped this information will ease the burden of the difficult choices that have to be made in the children's treatment. Parents who are informed can integrate their preferences with the safety and efficacy of a range of therapies and in this way can become powerful members of their child's treatment team.

Psychosocial and pharmacological interventions have traditionally been examined in separate studies with distinct differences in methods and designs, making it difficult to compare the relative efficacy and safety of these two modalities. This is a major limitation because treatment guidelines need to integrate all effective interventions—psychological, psychopharmacological, and combination. Also, the standards applied to these modalities should be comparable. As one step in this direction, a number of recent federally funded initiatives have directly compared the relative effectiveness of psychosocial and psychopharmacological interventions, alone and in combination (e.g., Multimodal Treatment of ADHD, Treatments for Adolescents With Depression Study, Pediatric OCD Treatment Study, and Child/Adolescent Anxiety Multimodal Treatment Study). These studies have their own limitations, but they offer additional perspectives on comparing treatments for children and adolescents.

A few general trends emerged from the literature reviewed for this report. Most notable, the evidence base for treatment efficacy is somewhat uneven across disorders, with most of the research focusing on childhood ADHD, adolescent depression, and more recently, anxiety disorders. Some of the most severe mental health conditions of childhood, including bipolar disorder and schizophrenia, have received proportionally less attention from treatment researchers. The use of psychosocial treatments as first-line interventions is supported for a number of conditions, including ADHD, oppositional defiant disorder, conduct disorder (CD), autism, anorexia nervosa and bulimia nervosa, obsessive–compulsive disorder (OCD), posttraumatic stress disorder (PTSD), other anxiety disorders, and depression. Psychosocial interventions, psychopharmacological interventions, or their combinations are effective, at least acutely for a number of disorders. These include ADHD and depression.

Despite recent advances in treatment research, wide knowledge gaps remain. Most of the evidence for efficacy is limited to acute symptom improvement, with only limited attention paid to functional outcomes and long-term effects. In addition, few studies have been conducted in practice settings and, with the possible exception of ADHD and CD, for which much research has been conducted in schools, little is known about the therapeutic benefits of intervention under real-life conditions. Furthermore, whereas the benefits of some behavioral treatments have been well documented through numerous single-subject design studies and group-crossover designs, there is a relative meager number of well-controlled, randomized clinical trials supporting their effectiveness.

Certain design features, including inadequate statistical power, choice of control group, and lack of an intent-to-treat analytical strategy, also limit the interpretation of research for a number of disorders. Few studies have addressed which treatment alternatives should occur first. Little empirical evidence is available to guide the management of initial treatment nonresponders. Many more studies need to investigate the sequencing and integration of different interventions, and more research should consider the high rates of diagnostic comorbidity in childhood, because few studies have addressed the treatment of youngsters with multiple disorders or other complex conditions.

For this book, as mentioned in chapter 1, the premise of *evidence-based practice* was defined as that set forth in the Institute of Medicine (2001) report: practice that "involves the integration of best research evidence with clinical expertise and patient values" (p. 145). We recognized this is a narrow definition of evidence-based practice but agreed to apply a narrower model to meet the charge of conducting a consistent, comparative analysis of psychotropic medications relative to psychosocial interventions. We noted our method is in concert with the American Psychological Association's (APA; 2005) *Policy Statement on Evidence-Based Practice in Psychology*. We relied on the best available evidence in scientific literature and reported the best evidence available for each major class of child and adolescent disorders.

A notable advance in the field has been the attempt to develop evidence-based clinical practice guidelines for a number of disorders, including ADHD, depression, OCD, bipolar disorder, and schizophrenia. Such guidelines represent an important step in translating research findings into practice, but the effort has been hampered by the current limitations in knowledge and research and by differences in the standards that are used to develop guidelines (e.g., summaries of evidence, expert consensus, guild consensus). In summary, great strides have been made in the development of beneficial treatments for child and adolescent mental health disorders, but significant gaps remain.

RESEARCH AND FUNDING

The development and dissemination of evidence-based treatments for child and adolescent psychopathology is a national priority (APA, 2003; U.S. Public Health Service, 2000). The notable gaps in our knowledge at this time are of great concern. The evidence base for treatments is uneven across disorders, age groups, and other defining characteristics (e.g., race, ethnicity, and socioeconomic status). Data are lacking on the long-term effects for most treatments and for their effects on functional outcomes (e.g., academic achievement, peer relationships). Pharmaceutical data not always being made available to the public has been a barrier to the understanding of efficacious treatments and possible associated adverse side effects, and especially to the trust relationship between providers and consumers. To advance knowledge in the field and improve the lives of children and adolescents and their families, researchers, research funding organizations, and other stakeholders, including those who establish funding priorities, must work together to strengthen the evidence base for the treatment of child and adolescent psychopathology. Mental health care practitioners need to apply additional attention to ways to improve communication, education, and trust, with consumers as treatment team members.

Several research priorities were revealed in the process of producing this book. Investigations of treatment efficacy, effectiveness, and safety should be conducted with several goals in mind: to examine outcomes in terms of symptoms, functional impairments, adaptive functioning, safety, and quality of life; to determine effect across groups from diverse backgrounds; and to focus on understudied age groups for each type of disorder where necessary (e.g., prepubertal depression, preschool and adolescent ADHD, adolescent autism). More research is also needed to determine optimal doses, intensities, compositions, and duration of psychosocial and psychopharmacological treatments. Researchers need to focus on optimal sequencing of multimodal treatment components that maximizes efficacy, including functional outcomes, and that minimizes adverse side effects. The differential contributions (both benefits and risks) of individual components in multicomponent treatments (e.g., combined psychosocial and psychopharmacological treatments and polypharmacy) must also be studied.

It is imperative that practitioners understand factors such as child and adolescent attitudes, parent preference, external barriers to treatment, and medication side effects, because they are all associated with efficacy of treatment. It is also incumbent on us as mental health care providers to understand the ways in which factors of diversity, including race and ethnicity, gender, sexual orientation, and disability, contribute to beliefs and attitudes about psychotropic drug use and engagement in treatment in general. Researchers must investigate the impact of systems-level factors (e.g., family structure and organization and financing) on evidence-based treatments for child and adolescent disorders. The cost-effectiveness of mental health services, especially contrasting the evidence-based practices of different modalities, doses, and types, sorely needs examination.

To facilitate research funding and the dissemination of outcomes, collaboration and sustained partnerships must be established in federal, private, and public sectors, including federal funding agencies involved in child treatment research (e.g., National Institute of Mental Health, National Institute of Child Health and Human Development, National Institute of Neurological Disorders and Stroke, Agency for Healthcare Research and Quality, Centers for Disease Control and Prevention, Substance Abuse and Mental Health Services Administration, and Institute of Education Sciences) and between private, professional, and public organizations. In addition, ongoing communication should become the norm among researchers, clinical providers, and families to facilitate the use of evidence-based practice in real-world settings.

To address issues of safety, all efficacy and safety data emanating from psychosocial and psychopharmacological treatment research on child and adolescent disorders should be released to the public. Federal monitoring agencies (e.g., the U.S. Food and Drug Administration) should be fully independent of political and economic influences. A governmental entity analogous to the U.S. Food and Drug Administration that monitors the development and marketing of psychosocial treatments should be established to serve the public.

PROFESSIONAL EDUCATION

In child and adolescent psychology, contemporary training in evidence-based interventions at the predoctoral, postdoctoral, and continuing education levels is essential. Psychosocial and psychopharmacological evidence-based treatments for childhood disorders must be a part of all curricula for applied psychologists working with children and families. Regardless of discipline, a working knowledge of current psychopharmacology and psychosocial therapies is paramount for all professionals involved in the treatment of child and adolescent disorders. In-depth multicultural competence training should be mandated in all preservice and in-service settings.

To become familiar with psychological interventions and develop skills in the implementation of psychosocial interventions for a variety of disorders, predoctoral training of professional psychologists must include a broad-based education in the various evidence-based treatments discussed in this book. Predoctoral students must receive training that renders them proficient in the critical review of treatment literature, which will ensure the ongoing review of and familiarity with the changes that will occur in the field during their careers. Training should include principles of clinical psychopharmacology and knowledge of current literature on pharmacological treatment efficacy. Coursework, training practica, and internships should include skill development in the procedures and instruments that are evidence based for monitoring client and patient outcomes in both clinical practice and clinical trials, including symptom change, functional outcomes (both positive and negative), and adverse side effects.

Training at the postdoctoral level must be organized to further the development of skills in the implementation of evidence-based psychosocial interventions and general knowledge of evidence-based psychopharmacological and psychosocial treatments, consistent with current training guidelines for postdoctoral fellowships for child and adolescent psychology. Educators should encourage postdoctoral fellows to continue the breadth and further increase the depth of training in evidence-based interventions.

Continuing education for child and adolescent practitioners and training faculty must emphasize contemporary evidence-based strategies in the treatment and management of childhood disorders. Practitioners must be taught systematic methods for monitoring medication and psychosocial treatment efficacy, and especially the evaluation of potential adverse side effects and functional outcomes. Collaboration with other treatment team members, including physicians, school personnel, caregivers, and others involved in the comprehensive care of youths (e.g., tutors, parole officers, case managers), is essential. In addition, providers must be taught to develop treatment plans and discuss risk–benefit analyses collaboratively with parents, adolescents, and sometimes children to facilitate informed decision making for treatment plans.

PUBLIC EDUCATION

A tremendous amount of information about childhood psychopathology and treatment is easily accessible from different sources, the most notable one being the Internet. Many parents, children, and family members use the World Wide Web to understand problems and treatments. Unfortunately, the quality and veracity of this information are highly variable and potentially misleading to consumers. In addition, media portrayals of mental illness in childhood and its treatment are at times inaccurate and misleading. Parents, caregivers, and others involved must be provided with accurate information about childhood mental health disorders and their efficacious treatment. To improve recognition and understanding of childhood mental illness and its treatment, professional organizations, the medical community, federal agencies, foundations, private industry, health care organizations, accrediting bodies, and others must commit to educating the public about these disorders and appropriate treatments that have been empirically demonstrated to have relative safety and efficacy.

To be informed choicemakers, parents and other consumers must be able to access accurate information about evidence-based treatments for child and adolescent mental health disorders. They need information on the benefits and risks of various psychosocial and psychotropic treatments and their influence on the functional problems for which the patients are being treated. These include information about treatments that do not work so the influence of "professionals" who make false or unsubstantiated claims about treatment effectiveness will be minimized. Practitioners must recognize that even the most educated and well-meaning parents can become naïve, hopeful consumers when their children's health is concerned. The media should be educated and encouraged to portray children and adolescents with mental health disorders accurately and to describe the evidence-based treatments they receive in a language style for the general public.

SERVICE DELIVERY

Our book did not address access and service delivery issues, but these clearly affect the ability to obtain safe, evidence-based, and effective treatments. Of youths identified with mental health disorders, at least 60% do not receive care, and many of those who do receive care see providers with limited or no expertise in pediatric mental health (U.S. Public Health Service, 2000).

The limited availability of providers trained in evidence-based treatments for child and adolescent mental health disorders underscores the critical importance of addressing not only the issues but also the best ways for consumers to access care. The development of an adequately trained workforce to disseminate evidence-based treatments as knowledge continues to develop will be crucial. New challenges must be addressed, for example, the need for continuing caution in the use of new medications, especially in light of the fact that 20% of new medications receive black box warnings or are removed from the market (Lasser et al., 2002). For youths and their families, the barriers to care may be many, including poor to no health insurance, transportation problems, and disparities between urban versus rural communities. Disparities in the use of mental health services by children and adolescents have also been noted along lines of race and ethnicity, socioeconomic status, gender, geographic regions, provider type, and physical disability (U.S. Public Health Service, 2000).

To address these issues, third-party carriers must establish systematic reimbursement for evidence-based psychosocial and psychopharmacological treatments. Current funding and administrative mechanisms often encourage the use of medication or non-evidence-based psychosocial treatments instead of empirically based and physically less intrusive psychosocial treatments. Mental health services for youths are provided across a number of different service sectors, either simultaneously or sequentially, and collaborative care is often hampered by cost, discipline, and administrative barriers. Policymakers, professional organizations, educational and training institutions, and providers must develop policy and implement practices ensuring that youths with mental health disorders are identified and have access to empirically validated, safe, reimbursable treatments. These efforts should include parents, children, and families on panels formed to improve access to care.

As knowledge continues to develop, public policy efforts must establish an ongoing mechanism to disseminate scientifically proven information on the benefits and risks of psychosocial and psychopharmacological interventions and facilitate their implementation. Advocacy should focus on the establishment of partnerships among government funding agencies at the federal, state, and local levels, large insurers and managed care organizations, and regulatory bodies to allow private and public mental health agencies to develop a workforce of providers trained in evidence-based practice. Partnerships, particularly interdisciplinary partnerships among physicians, mental health practitioners, educators and schools, community leaders, government agencies, and families, should be developed to ensure adaptation, dissemination, and implementation of evidence-based treatments.

Access to and coordination of quality mental health care services at the local, state, and national levels are especially salient issues. Where data suggest that youths are receiving substandard or more risky care because of lack of access, practitioners must work to change the health and mental health care delivery systems and challenge any roadblocks to change. Collaborative care models should be developed, both fiscally and administratively, that provide mental health services for children and adolescents in a variety of settings through a number of public and private mechanisms, including, but not limited to, subspecialty mental health, primary care, schools, child welfare and child protective services, and juvenile justice.

Collaborative decision making should be promoted to the norm among providers, parents, and youths so that careful risk–benefit analyses and informed treatment planning are accomplished. Care should be delivered in a family-focused, culturally competent manner that encompasses child and family preferences and values in treatment choices. Given the potential harm of psychotropic drugs, the lack of data on safety of drug combinations, and lack of long-term data on safety, practitioners should be encouraged first to consider successful nonpsychopharmacological treatments when appropriate. If medication is seen as necessary, then providers should be encouraged to treat youths with the lowest dose and fewest number of appropriate medications and for the shortest possible time period. Clinicians must be supported in their role as advocates for improved and effective mental health care for children and adolescents.

CONCLUSION

Over the past several years, a number of important developments have been made with psychosocial and psychopharmacological treatments for children and adolescents with mental health disorders. Critical issues have emerged, including the safety and efficacy of various psychopharmacological and psychosocial treatments when used either alone or in combination. Throughout this book, our review and analysis posed a number of important questions for future research efforts, and several policy issues emerged that if resolved we hope will have an effect on mental health service delivery issues. It is our hope that these efforts will stimulate future research and policy as well as ultimately enhance the quality of life for children and adolescents with mental health disorders and their families.

REFERENCES

Abikoff, H., Hechtman, L., Klein, R. G., Weiss, G., Fleiss, K., Etcovitch, J., et al. (2004). Symptomatic improvement in children with ADHD treated with long-term methylphenidate and multimodal psychosocial treatment. *Journal of the American Academy of Child & Adolescent Psychiatry, 43*, 802–811.

Abramowitz, A. J., Eckstrand, D., O'Leary, S. G., & Dulcan, M. K. (1992). ADHD children's responses to stimulant medication and two intensities of a behavioral intervention. *Behavior Modification, 16*, 193–203.

Abramowitz, J. S. (1997). Effectiveness of psychological and pharmacological treatments for obsessive–compulsive disorder: A quantitative review. *Journal of Consulting and Clinical Psychology, 65*, 44–52.

Abramowitz, J. S., Whiteside, S., & Deacon, B. (2005). The effectiveness of treatment for pediatric obsessive–compulsive disorder: A meta-analysis. *Behavior Therapy, 36*, 55–63.

Achenbach, T. M., Howell, C. T., McConaughy, S. H., & Stanger, C. (1995). Six-year predictors of problems in a national sample of children and youth: I. Cross-informant syndromes. *Journal of the American Academy of Child & Adolescent Psychiatry, 34*, 336–347.

Achenbach, T. M., Krukowski, R., Dumenci, L., & Ivanova, M. (2005). Assessment of adult psychopathology: Meta-analyses and implications of cross-informant correlations. *Psychological Bulletin, 131*, 361–382.

Achenbach, T. M., McConaughy, S. H., & Howell, C. T. (1987). Child/adolescent behavioral and emotional problems: Implications of cross-informant correlations for situational specificity. *Psychological Bulletin, 101*, 213–232.

Ackerson, J., Scogin, F., McKendree-Smith, N., & Lyman, R. D. (1998). Cognitive bibliotherapy for mild and moderate adolescent depressive symptomatology. *Journal of Consulting and Clinical Psychology, 66*, 685–690.

Aegisdóttir, S., White, M. J., & Spengler, P. M. (2006). The meta-analysis of clinical judgment project: Fifty-six years of accumulated research on clinical versus statistical prediction. *Counseling Psychologist, 34*, 341–382.

Akin-Little, K. A., Eckert, T. L., Lovett, B. J., & Little, S. G. (2004). Extrinsic reinforcement in the classroom: Bribery or best practice. *School Psychology Review, 33*, 344–362.

Aman, M. G., Arnold, L. E., & Armstrong, S. C. (1999). Review of serotonergic agents and perseverative behavior in patients with developmental disabilities. *Mental Retardation and Developmental Disabilities Research Reviews, 5*, 279–289.

Aman, M. G., Lam, K. S., & Collier-Crespin, A. (2003). Prevalence and patterns of use of psychotropic medicines among individuals with autism in the Autism Society of Ohio. *Journal of Autism and Developmental Disorders, 33*, 527–534.

Aman, M. G., Lam, K. S., & Van Bourgondien, M. E. (2005). Medication patterns in patients with autism: Temporal, regional, and demographic influences. *Journal of Child and Adolescent Psychopharmacology, 15*, 116–126.

Aman, M. G., & Lindsay, R. L. (2002, October). Psychotropic medicines and aggressive behavior: Part I. Psychostimulants. *Child and Adolescent Psychopharmacology News, 7*(5), 1–6.

Ambrosini, P. J., Bianchi, M. D., Rabinovich, H., & Elia, J. (1993). Antidepressant treatment in children and adolescents: I. Affective disorders. *Journal of the American Academy of Child & Adolescent Psychiatry, 32*, 1–6.

American Academy of Child & Adolescent Psychiatry. (2002). Practice parameter for the use of stimulant medications in the treatment of children, adolescents, and adults. *Journal of the American Academy of Child & Adolescent Psychiatry, 41*(Suppl. 2), 26S–49S.

American Academy of Pediatrics. (2001a). Clinical practice guideline: Diagnosis and evaluation of a child with attention-deficit/hyperactivity disorder. *Pediatrics, 105*, 1158–1170.

American Academy of Pediatrics. (2001b). Clinical practice guideline: Treatment of the school-aged child with attention-deficit/hyperactivity disorder. *Pediatrics, 105*, 1033–1038.

American Diabetes Association, American Psychiatric Association, American Association of Clinical Endocrinologists, & North American Association for the Study of Obesity. (2004). Consensus development conference on antipsychotic drugs and obesity and diabetes. *Obesity Research, 12*, 362–368.

American Psychiatric Association. (2000). *Diagnostic and statistical manual of mental disorders* (4th ed., text rev.). Washington, DC: Author.

American Psychological Association. (2002). Ethical principles of psychologists and code of conduct. *American Psychologist, 57*, 1060–1073; also available at http://www.apa.org/ethics/code2002.html

American Psychological Association. (2003). *APA resolution on children's mental health*. Retrieved May 25, 2005, from http://www.apa.org/pi/resolution/childmentalhlth.html

American Psychological Association. (2005). *Policy statement on evidence-based practice in psychology*. Retrieved May 30, 2005, from http://www2.apa.org/practice/ebpstatement.pdf

Anastopoulos, A. D., Shelton, T. L., & Barkley, R. A. (2005). Family-based psychosocial treatments for children and adolescents with attention-deficit/hyperactivity disorder. In E. D. Hibbs & P. S. Jensen (Eds.), *Psychosocial treatments for child and adolescent disorders: Empirically based strategies for clinical practice* (pp. 327–350). Washington, DC: American Psychological Association.

Anastopoulos, A. D., Shelton, T. L., DuPaul, G. J., & Guevremont, D. C. (1993). Parent training for attention-deficit hyperactivity disorder: Its impact on parent functioning. *Journal of Abnormal Child Psychology, 21*, 581–596.

Anderson, C. M., Griffin, S., Rossi, A., Pagonis, I., Holder, D. P., & Treiber, R. (1986). A comparative study of the impact of education vs. process groups for families of patients with affective disorders. *Family Process, 25*, 185–205.

Anderson, D. A., & Maloney, K. C. (2001). The efficacy of cognitive–behavioral therapy on the core symptoms of bulimia nervosa. *Clinical Psychology Review, 21*, 971–988.

Anderson, L. T., Campbell, M., Adams, P., Small, A. M., Perry, R., & Shell, J. (1989). The effects of haloperidol on discrimination learning and behavioral symptoms in autistic children. *Journal of Autism and Developmental Disorders, 19*, 227–239.

Anderson, S. L., Arvanitogiannis, A., Pliakas, A., LeBlanc, C., & Carlezon, W. (2002). Altered responsiveness to cocaine in rats exposed to methylphenidate during development. *Nature Neuroscience, 5*, 13–14.

Ansorge, M. S., Zhou, M., Lira, A., Hen, R., & Gingrich, J. A. (2004, October 29). Early-life blockade of the 5-HT transporter alters emotional behavior in adult mice. *Science, 306*, 879–881.

Antonuccio, D. O., Danton, W. G., DeNelsky, G. Y., Greenberg, R. P., & Gordon, J. S. (1999). Raising questions about antidepressants. *Psychotherapy and Psychosomatics, 68*, 3–14.

Antonuccio, D. O., Danton, W. G., & McClanahan, T. M. (2003). Psychology in the prescription era: Building a firewall between marketing and science. *American Psychologist, 58*, 1028–1043.

Antonuccio, D. O., Thomas, M., & Danton, W. G. (1997). A cost-effectiveness analysis of cognitive behavior therapy and fluoxetine (Prozac) in the treatment of depression. *Behavior Therapy, 28*, 187–210.

Arnold, A. L., Elliott, M., Sachs, L., Bird, H., Kraemer, H. C., Wells, K. C., et al. (2003). Effects of ethnicity on treatment attendance, stimulant response/dose, and 14-month outcome in ADHD. *Journal of Consulting and Clinical Psychology, 71*, 713–727.

Asarnow, J. R., Jaycox, L. H., Duan, N., LaBorde, A., Guthrie, D., & Wells, K. B. (2003, September). *Depression among adolescents in primary care: Youth partners in care*. Paper presented at the annual meeting of the Child Depression Consortium, Pittsburgh, PA.

Asarnow, J. R., Jaycox, L. H., Duan, N., LaBorde, A. P., Rea, M. M., Murray, P., et al. (2005). Effectiveness of a quality improvement intervention for adolescent depression in primary care clinics: A randomized controlled trial. *Journal of the American Medical Association, 293*, 311–319.

Asarnow, J. R., & Tompson, M. C. (1999). Childhood-onset schizophrenia: A follow-up study. *European Child and Adolescent Psychiatry, 8*(Suppl.), 19–12.

Asarnow, J. R., Tompson, M. C., & McGrath, E. (2004). Annotation: Childhood-onset schizophrenia: Clinical and treatment issues. *Journal of Child Psychology and Psychiatry, 45*, 180–194.

Azrin, N. H., & Nunn, R. G. (1973). Habit reversal: A method of eliminating nervous habits and tics. *Behavior Research and Therapy, 11*, 619–628.

Azrin, N. H., & Peterson, A. L. (1990). Treatment of Tourette syndrome by habit reversal: A waiting-list control group comparison. *Behavior Therapy, 21*, 305–318.

Bacaltchuk, J., Hay, P., & Mari, J. J. (2000). Antidepressants versus placebo for the treatment of bulimia nervosa: A systematic review. *Australian and New Zealand Journal of Psychiatry, 34,* 310–317.

Bahl, S., Cotterchio, M., & Kreiger, N. (2003). Use of antidepressant medications and the possible association with breast cancer risk: A review. *Psychotherapy and Psychosomatics, 72,* 185–194.

Baldessarini, R. J. (1995). Risks and implications of interrupting maintenance psychotropic drug therapy. *Psychotherapy and Psychosomatics, 63,* 137–141.

Barbarich, N. C., McConaha, C. W., Gaskill, J., La Via, M., Frank, G. F., Achenbach, S., et al. (2004). An open trial of olanzapine in anorexia nervosa. *Journal of Clinical Psychiatry, 65,* 1480–1482.

Barkley, R. A. (1988). The effects of methylphenidate on the interactions of preschool ADHD children with their mothers. *Journal of the American Academy of Child & Adolescent Psychiatry, 27,* 336–341.

Barkley, R. A. (2003). Issues in the diagnosis of attention-deficit/hyperactivity disorder in children. *Brain & Development, 25,* 77–83.

Barkley, R. A., Edwards, G., Laneri, M., Fletcher, K., & Metevia, L. (2001). The efficacy of problem-solving communication training alone, behavior management training alone, and their combination for parent–adolescent conflict in teenagers with ADHD and ODD. *Journal of Consulting and Clinical Psychology, 69,* 926–941.

Barkley, R. A., & Fischer, M. (2005). Suicidality in children with ADHD. *The ADHD Report, 13*(6), 1–4.

Barkley, R. A., Fischer, M., Smallish, L., & Fletcher, K. (2003). Does the treatment of attention-deficit/hyperactivity disorder with stimulants contribute to drug use/abuse? A 13-year prospective study. *Pediatrics, 111,* 97–109.

Barkley, R. A., Shelton, T. L., Crosswait, C., Moorehouse, M., Fletcher, K., Barrett, S., et al. (2000). Multi-method psycho-educational intervention for preschool children with disruptive behavior: Preliminary results at post-treatment. *Journal of Child Psychology and Psychiatry and Allied Disciplines, 41,* 319–332.

Barmish, A. J., & Kendall, P. C. (2005). Should parents be co-clients in cognitive–behavioral therapy for anxious youth? *Journal of Clinical Child and Adolescent Psychology, 34,* 569–581.

Barrett, P., Dadds, M., & Rapee, R. (1996). Family treatment of childhood anxiety: A controlled trial. *Journal of Consulting and Clinical Psychology, 64,* 333–342.

Barrett, P., Duffy, A., Dadds, M., & Rapee, R. (2001). Cognitive–behavioral treatment of anxiety disorders in children: Long-term (6-year) follow-up. *Journal of Consulting and Clinical Psychology, 69,* 135–141.

Barrett, P., Healy-Farrell, L., & March, J. (2004). Cognitive–behavioral family treatment of childhood obsessive–compulsive disorder: A controlled trial. *Journal of the American Academy of Child & Adolescent Psychiatry, 43,* 46–62.

Bauman, L. (2000). A patient-centered approach to adherence: Risks for nonadherence. In D. Drotar (Ed.), *Promoting adherence to medical treatment in chronic childhood illness: Concepts, methods, and interventions* (pp. 71–93). New York: Erlbaum.

Baumeister, A. A., & Baumeister, A. A. (1995). Mental retardation. In M. Hersen & R. L. Ammerman (Eds.), *Advanced abnormal child psychology* (pp. 283–303). Hillsdale, NJ: Erlbaum.

Begg, C. B., Cho, M. K., Eastwood, S., Horton, R., Moher, D., Olkin, I., et al. (1996). Improving the quality of reporting of randomized controlled trials: The CONSORT statement. *Journal of the American Medical Association, 276*, 637–639.

Beidel, D. C., Turner, S. M., & Morris, T. L. (2000). Behavioral treatment of childhood social phobia. *Journal of Consulting and Clinical Psychology, 68*, 1072–1080.

Benjamin, R. S., Costello, E. J., & Warren, M. (1990). Anxiety disorders in a pediatric sample. *Journal of Anxiety Disorders, 4*, 293–316.

Bergman, R. L., & Piacentini, J. (2005). Selective mutism. In H. Kaplan & B. Sadock (Eds.), *Comprehensive textbook of psychiatry* (8th ed., pp. 3302–3306). Philadelphia: Lippincott Williams & Wilkins.

Bernstein, G. A., Borchardt, C. M., Perwien, A. R., Crosby, R. D., Kushner, M. G., Thuras, P. D., & Last, C. G. (2000). Imipramine plus cognitive–behavioral therapy in the treatment of school refusal. *Journal of the American Academy of Child & Adolescent Psychiatry, 39*, 276–283.

Biederman, J., Kwon, A., Wozniak, J., Mick, E., Markowitz, S., Fazio, V., & Faraone, S. V. (2004). Absence of gender differences in pediatric bipolar disorder: Findings from a large sample of referred youth. *Journal of Affective Disorders, 83*(2–3), 207–214.

Biederman, J., Lopez, F. A., Boellner, S. W., & Chandler, M. C. (2002). A randomized, double-blind, placebo-controlled, parallel-group study of SLI381 (Adderall XR) in children with attention-deficit/hyperactivity disorder. *Pediatrics, 110*, 258–266.

Biederman, J., Wilens, T., Mick, E., Spencer, T., & Faraone, S. V. (1999). Pharmacotherapy of attention-deficit/hyperactivity disorder reduces risk for substance use disorder. *Pediatrics, 104*, e20.

Birmaher, B., Axelson, D. A., Monk, K., Kalas, C., Clark, D. B., Ehmann, M., et al. (2003). Fluoxetine for the treatment of childhood anxiety disorders. *Journal of the American Academy of Child & Adolescent Psychiatry, 42*, 415–423.

Birmaher, B., Brent, D. A., Kolko, D., Baugher, M., Bridge, J., Holder, D., et al. (2000). Clinical outcome after short-term psychotherapy for adolescents with major depressive disorder. *Archives of General Psychiatry, 57*, 29–36.

Black, B., & Uhde, T. (1994). Treatment of elective mutism with fluoxetine: A double-blind, placebo-controlled study. *Journal of the American Academy of Child & Adolescent Psychiatry, 33*, 1000–1006.

Bor, W., Sanders, M. R., & Markie-Dadds, C. (2002). The effects of the Triple-P Positive Parenting Program on preschool children with co-occurring disruptive behavior and attention/hyperactive difficulties. *Journal of Abnormal Child Psychology, 30*, 571–587.

Bower, P. (2003). Efficacy in evidence-based practice. *Clinical Psychology and Psychotherapy, 10*, 328–336.

Brent, D. A. (2004). Antidepressants and pediatric depression: The risk of doing nothing. *New England Journal of Medicine, 351*, 1598–601.

Brent, D. A., Holder, D., Kolko, D., Birmaher, B., Baugher, M., Roth, C., et al. (1997). A clinical psychotherapy trial for adolescent depression comparing cognitive, family, and supportive therapy. *Archives of General Psychiatry, 54*, 877–885.

Brent, D. A., Kolko, D. J., Birmaher, B., Baugher, M., & Bridge, J. (1999). A clinical trial for adolescent depression: Predictors of additional treatment in the acute and follow-up phases of the trial. *Journal of the American Academy of Child & Adolescent Psychiatry*, 38, 263–270.

Brent, D. A., Poling, K., McKain, B., & Baugher, M. (1993). A psychoeducational program for families of affectively ill children and adolescents. *Journal of the American Academy of Child & Adolescent Psychiatry, 32*, 770–774.

Brestan, E. V., & Eyberg, S. M. (1998). Effective psychosocial treatments of conduct-disordered children and adolescents: 29 years, 82 studies, and 5272 kids. *Journal of Clinical Child Psychology, 27*, 180–189.

Bridge, J. A., Iyengar, S., Salary, C. B., Barbe, R. P., Birmaher, B., Pincus, H. A., et al. (2007). Clinical response and risk for reported suicidal ideation and suicide attempts in pediatric antidepressant treatment: A meta-analysis of randomized controlled trials. *Journal of the American Medical Association, 297*, 1683–1696.

Brown, G. K., Ten Have, T., Henriques, G. R., Xie, S. X., Hollander, J. E., & Beck, A. T. (2005). Cognitive therapy for the prevention of suicide attempts: A randomized controlled trial. *Journal of the American Medical Association, 294*, 563–570.

Brown, R. T., & Daly, B. (in press). Neuropsychological effects of stimulant medication on children's learning and behavior. In C. R. Reynolds & E. Fletcher-Jantzen (Eds.), *Handbook of clinical child neuropsychology* (3rd ed.). New York: Springer Publishing Company.

Brown, R. T., Daly, B., & Rickel (2007). *Chronic illness in children and adolescents.* Cambridge, MA: Hogrefe & Huber.

Brown, R. T., & Sammons, M. T. (2002). Pediatric psychopharmacology: A review of new developments and recent research. *Professional Psychology: Research and Practice, 33*, 135–147.

Brown, R. T., & Sawyer, M. G. (1998). *Medications for school-age children: Effects on and learning and behavior.* New York: Guilford Press.

Brown, R. T., & Sexson, S. B. (1987). A controlled trial of methylphenidate in Black adolescents. *Clinical Pediatrics, 27*, 74–81.

Brown, R. T. & Zygmont, D. (in press). Psychopharmacology. In T. B. Gutkin & C. R. Reynolds (Eds.), *The handbook of school psychology* (4th ed.). New York: Wiley.

Brown, T .E. (2004). Atomoxetine and stimulants in combination for treatment of attention deficit hyperactivity disorder: Four case reports. *Journal of Child and Adolescent Psychopharmacology, 14*, 129–136.

Bryson, S. E., Rogers, S. J., & Fombonne, E. (2003). Autism spectrum disorders: Early detection, intervention, education, and psychopharmacological management. *Canadian Journal of Psychiatry, 48*, 506–516.

Burns, B. J., Costello, E. J., Angold, A., Tweed, D., Stangl, D., Farmer, E. M., & Erkanli, A. (1995). Children's mental health service use across service sectors. *Health Affairs, 14*, 147–159.

Bussing, R., Zima, B. T., Mason, D., Hou, W., Garvan, C. W., & Forness, S. (2005). Use and persistence of pharmacotherapy for elementary school students with attention-deficit/hyperactivity disorder. *Journal of Child and Adolescent Psychopharmacology, 15*, 78–87.

Butzlaff, R. L., & Hooley, J. M. (1998). Expressed emotion and psychiatric relapse. *Archives of General Psychiatry, 55*, 547–552.

Byrne, N., Regan, C., & Livingston, G. (2006). Adherence to treatment in mood disorders. *Current Opinion in Psychiatry, 19*, 44–49.

Campbell, M., Adams, P., Small, A. M., Curren, E. L., Overall, J. E., Anderson, L. T., et al. (1988). Efficacy and safety of fenfluramine in autistic children. *Journal of the American Academy of Child & Adolescent Psychiatry, 27*, 434–439.

Campbell, M., Armenteros, J. L., Malone, R. P., Adams, P., Eisenberg, Z. W., & Overall, J. E. (1997). Neuroleptic-related dyskinesias in autistic children: A prospective, longitudinal study. *Journal of the American Academy of Child & Adolescent Psychiatry, 36*, 835–843.

Campbell, M., Cohen, I. L., & Small, A. M. (1982). Drugs in aggressive behavior. *Journal of the American Academy of Child Psychiatry, 21*, 107–117.

Carlson, G. L., Pelham, W. E., Milich, R., & Dixon, M. J. (1992). Single and combined effects of methylphenidate and behavior therapy on the classroom behavior, academic performance and self-evaluations of children with attention-deficit hyperactivity disorder. *Journal of Abnormal Child Psychology, 20*, 213–232.

Cartwright-Hatton, S., Roberts, C., Chitsabesan, P., Fothergill, C., & Harrington, R. (2004). Systematic review of the efficacy of cognitive behaviour therapies for childhood and adolescent anxiety disorders. *British Journal of Clinical Psychology*, 43, 421–436.

Casat, C. D., Pleasants, D. Z., Schroeder, D. H., & Parker, D. W. (1989). Bupropion in children with attention deficit disorder. *Psychopharmacology Bulletin, 25*, 198–201.

Centers for Disease Control and Prevention. (2004). *National Center for Health Statistics: National health interview survey*. Washington, DC: Author.

Chacko, A., Pelham, W. E., Gnagy, E. M., Greiner, A., Vallano, G., Bukstein, O., & Rancurello, M. (2005). Stimulant medication effects in a natural setting among young children with attention-deficit/hyperactivity disorder. *Journal of the American Academy of Child & Adolescent Psychiatry, 4*, 249–257.

Chakrabarti, S., & Fombonne, E. (2005). Pervasive developmental disorders in preschool children: Confirmation of high prevalence. *American Journal of Psychiatry, 162*, 1133–1141.

Chamberlain, P., Fisher, P. A., & Moore, K. (2002). Multidimensional treatment foster care: Applications of the OSLC intervention model to high-risk youth and their families. In J. B. Reid, G. R. Patterson, & J. Snyder (Eds.), *Antisocial behavior in children and adolescents: A developmental analysis and model for intervention* (pp. 203–218). Washington, DC: American Psychological Association.

Cheng-Shannon, J., McGough, J., Pataki, C., & McCracken, J. (2004). Second-generation antipsychotic medications in children and adolescents. *Journal of Child and Adolescent Psychopharmacology, 14*, 372–394.

Chilvers, C., Dewey, M., Fielding, K., Gretton, V., Miller, P., Palmer, B., et al. (2001). Antidepressant drugs and generic counseling for treatment of major depression in primary care: Randomised trial with patient preference arms. *British Medical Journal, 322*, 772–775.

Christman, A. K., Fermo, J. D., & Markowitz, J. S. (2004). Atomoxetine, a novel treatment for attention-deficit-hyperactivity disorder. *Pharmacotherapy, 24*, 1020–1036.

Chronis, A. M., Fabiano, G. A., Gnagy, E. M., Onyango, A. N., Pelham, W. E., Williams, A., et al. (2004). An evaluation of the summer treatment program for children with attention-deficit/hyperactivity disorder using a treatment withdrawal design. *Behavior Therapy, 35*, 561–585.

Clarke, G. N., Rohde, P., Lewinsohn, P. M., Hops, H., & Seeley, J. R. (1999). Cognitive–behavioral treatment of adolescent depression: Efficacy of acute group treatment and booster sessions. *Journal of the American Academy of Child & Adolescent Psychiatry, 38*, 272–279.

Cobham, V. E., Dadds, M. R., & Spence, S. H. (1998). The role of parental anxiety in the treatment of childhood anxiety. *Journal of Consulting and Clinical Psychology, 66*, 893–905.

Cohen, J. (1988). *Statistical power analysis for the behavioral sciences* (2nd ed.). Hillsdale, NJ: Erlbaum.

Cohen, J. A., Deblinger, E., Mannarino, A. P., & Steer, R. A. (2004). A multisite, randomized controlled trial for children with sexual abuse-related PTSD symptoms. *Journal of the American Academy of Child & Adolescent Psychiatry, 43*, 393–402.

Cohn, L. M., & Caliendo, G. C. (1997). Guanfacine use in children with attention deficit hyperactivity disorder. *Annals of Pharmacotherapy, 31*, 918–919.

Compton, S. N., Burns, B. J., Egger, H. L., & Robertson, E. (2002). Review of the evidence base for treatment of childhood psychopathology: Internalizing disorders. *Journal of Consulting and Clinical Psychology, 70*, 1240–1266.

Compton, S. N., March, J. S., Brent, D., Albano, A. M., Weersing, V. R., & Curry, J. (2004). Cognitive–behavioral psychotherapy for anxiety and depressive disorders in children and adolescents: An evidence-based medicine review. *Journal of the American Academy of Child & Adolescent Psychiatry, 43*, 930–959.

Conners, C. K. (2002). Forty years of methylphenidate treatment in attention-deficit/hyperactivity disorder. *Journal of Attention Disorders*, 6(Suppl. 1), S17–S30.

Conners, C. K., Casat, C. D., Gualtieri, C. T., Weller, E., Reader, M., Reiss, A., et al. (1996). Bupropion hydrochloride in attention deficit disorder with hyperactivity. *Journal of the American Academy of Child & Adolescent Psychiatry, 35,* 1314–1321.

Conners, C. K., Epstein, J. N., March, J. S., Angold, A., Wells, K. C., Klaric, J., et al. (2001). Multimodal treatment of ADHD in the MTA: An alternative outcome analysis. *Journal of the American Academy of Child & Adolescent Psychiatry, 40,* 159–167.

Connor, D. F. (2005a). Other medications. In R. A. Barkley (Ed.), *Attention-deficit hyperactivity disorder: A handbook for diagnosis and treatment* (3rd ed., pp. 658–677). New York: Guilford Press.

Connor, D. F. (2005b). Stimulants. In R. A. Barkley (Ed.), *Attention-deficit hyperactivity disorder: A handbook for diagnosis and treatment* (3rd ed., pp. 608–647). New York: Guilford Press.

Connor, D. F., Fletcher, K. E., & Swanson, J. M. (1999). A meta-analysis of clonidine for symptoms of attention-deficit/hyperactivity disorder. *Journal of the American Academy of Child & Adolescent Psychiatry, 38,* 1551–1559.

Connor-Smith, J., & Weisz, J. (2003). Applying treatment outcome research in clinical practice: Techniques for adapting interventions to the real world. *Child and Adolescent Mental Health, 8,* 3–10.

Cook, E., Wagner, K., March, J., Biederman, J., Landau, P., Wolkow, R., & Messig, M. (2001). Long-term sertraline treatment of children and adolescents with obsessive–compulsive disorder. *Journal of the American Academy of Child & Adolescent Psychiatry, 40,* 1175–1181.

Costello, E. J., & Angold, A. (1995). Epidemiology. In J. March (Ed.), *Anxiety disorders in children and adolescents* (pp. 109–124). New York: Guilford Press.

Costello, E. J., Mustillo, S., Erkanli, A., Keeler, G., & Angold, A. (2003). Prevalence and development of psychiatric disorders in childhood and adolescence. *Archives of General Psychiatry, 60,* 837–844.

Cotgrove, A., Zirinsky, L., Black, D., & Weston, D. (1995). Secondary prevention of attempted suicide in adolescence. *Journal of Adolescence, 18,* 569–577.

Cotterchio, M., Kreiger, N., Darlington, G., & Steingart, A. (2000). Antidepressant medication use and breast cancer risk. *American Journal of Epidemiology, 151,* 951–957.

Coupland, N. J., Bell, C. J., & Potokar, J. P. (1996). Serotonin reuptake inhibitor withdrawal. *Journal of Clinical Psychopharmacology, 16,* 356–362.

Cox, D. J., Sutphen, J., Borowitz, S., Kovatchev, B., & Ling, W. (1998). Contribution of behavior therapy and biofeedback to laxative therapy in the treatment of pediatric encopresis. *Annals of Behavioral Medicine, 20,* 70–76.

Coyle, J. T., Pine, D. S., Charney, D. S., Lewis, L., Nemeroff, C. B., Carlson, G. A., et al. (2003). Depression and Bipolar Support Alliance Consensus Statement on the unmet needs in diagnosis and treatment of mood disorders in children and adolescents. *Journal of the American Academy of Child & Adolescent Psychiatry, 42,* 1494–1503.

Csoka, A. B., & Shipko, S. (2006). Persistent sexual side effects after SSRI discontinuation. *Psychotherapy and Psychosomatics, 75*, 187–188.

Cummings, D. D., Singer, H. S., Krieger, M., Miller, T. L., & Mahone, E. M. (2002). Neuropsychiatric effects of guanfacine in children with mild Tourette syndrome: A pilot study. *Clinical Neuropharmacology, 6*, 325–332.

Cunningham, C. E., & Cunningham, L. J. (1998). Student-mediated conflict resolution programs. In R. A. Barkley (Ed.), *Attention-deficit hyperactivity disorder: A handbook for diagnosis and treatment* (2nd ed., pp. 491–509). New York: Guilford Press.

Curry, J. F., & Wells, K. C. (2005). Striving for effectiveness in the treatment of adolescent depression. *Cognitive and Behavioral Practice, 12*, 177–185.

Dalfen, A. K., & Stewart, D. E. (2001). Who develops stable or fatal adverse drug reactions to selective serotonin reuptake inhibitors? *Canadian Journal of Psychiatry, 46*, 258–262.

Davis, T., & Ollendick, T. (2005). Empirically supported treatments for specific phobia in children: Do efficacious treatments address the components of a phobic response? *Clinical Psychology: Science and Practice, 12*, 144–160.

DeAngelis, C., Drazen, J. M., Frizelle, F. A., Haug, C., Hoey, J., Horton, R., et al. (2004). Clinical trial registration: A statement from the International Committee of Medical Journal Editors. *The Lancet, 364*, 911–912.

de Haan, E., Hoogduin, K. A., Buitelaar, J., & Keijsers, G. (1998). Behavior therapy versus clomipramine for the treatment of obsessive–compulsive disorder. *Journal of the American Academy of Child & Adolescent Psychiatry, 37*, 1022–1029.

DelBello, M. P., Schwiers, M. L., Rosenberg, H. L., & Strakowski, S. M. (2002). A double-blind, randomized, placebo-controlled study of quetiapine as adjunctive treatment for adolescent mania. *Journal of the American Academy of Child & Adolescent Psychiatry, 41*, 1216–1223.

Depressing research [Editorial]. (2004). *The Lancet, 363*, 1335.

Dishion, T. J., & Dodge, K. A. (2005). Peer contagion in interventions for children and adolescents: Moving towards an understanding of the ecology and dynamics of change. *Journal of Abnormal Child Psychology, 33*, 395–400.

Donovan, S., Madeley, R., Clayton, A., Beeharry, M., Jones, S., Kirk, C., et al. (2000). Deliberate self-harm and antidepressant drugs: Investigation of a possible link. *British Journal of Psychiatry, 177*, 551–556.

Doleys, D. M. (1977). Behavioral treatments for nocturnal enuresis in children: A review of the recent literature. *Psychological Bulletin, 84*, 30–54.

Drotar, D. (2006). *Psychological interventions in childhood chronic illness*. Washington, DC: American Psychological Association.

DuBois, D. L., Felner, R. D., Bartels, C. L., & Silverman, M. M. (1995). Stability of self-reported depressive symptoms in a community sample of children and adolescents. *Journal of Clinical Child Psychology, 4*, 386–396.

Dujovne, V. F., Barnard, M. U., & Rapoff, M. A. (1995). Pharmacological and cognitive–behavioral approaches in the treatment of childhood depression: A review and critique. *Clinical Psychology Review, 15*, 589–611.

Dunlap, G., dePerczel, M., Clarke, S., Wilson, D., Wright, S., White, R., & Gomez, A. (1994). Choice making to promote adaptive behavior for students with emotional and behavioral challenges. *Journal of Applied Behavior Analysis, 27,* 505–518.

DuPaul, G. J., & Eckert, T. L. (1997). The effects of school-based interventions for attention deficit hyperactivity disorder: A meta-analysis. *School Psychology Review, 26,* 5–27.

DuPaul, G. J., Ervin, R. A., Hook, C. L., & McGoey, K. E. (1998). Peer tutoring for children with attention deficit hyperactivity disorder: Effects on classroom behavior and academic performance. *Journal of Applied Behavior Analysis, 31,* 579–592.

DuPaul, G. J., Jitendra, A. K., Volpe, R. J., Lutz, J. G., Vile Junod, R., Tresco, K. E., et al. (2005, June). *Consultation-based academic interventions for children with ADHD: School functioning outcomes.* Poster presented at the biennial conference of the International Society for Research in Child and Adolescent Psychopathology, New York.

DuPaul, G. J., & Stoner, G. (2003). *ADHD in the schools: Assessment and intervention strategies.* New York: Guilford Press.

Eaton, W. W. (1995). Progress in the epidemiology of anxiety disorders. *Epidemiologic Reviews, 17,* 32–38.

Edwards, R. J., & Pople, I. K. (2002). Side-effects of risperidone therapy mimicking cerebrospinal fluid shunt malfunction: Implications for clinical monitoring and management. *Journal of Psychopharmacology, 16,* 177–179.

Eggers, C., Bunk, D., & Ropcke, B. (2002). Childhood and adolescent onset schizophrenia: Results from two long-term follow-up studies. *Neurology, Psychiatry and Brain Research,* 9, 183–190.

Eikeseth, S., Smith, T., Jahr, E., & Eldevik, S. (2002). Intensive behavioral treatment at school for 4- to 7-year-old children with autism: 1-year comparison controlled study. *Behavior Modification, 26,* 49–68.

Eisler, I., Dare, C., Hodes, M., Russell, G., Dodge, E., & LeGrange, D. (2000). Family therapy for adolescent anorexia nervosa: The results of a controlled comparison of two family interventions. *Journal of Child Psychology and Psychiatry, 41,* 727–736.

Emslie, G. J., Heiligenstein, J. H., Wagner, K. D., Hood, S. L., Ernest, D. E., Brown, E., et al. (2002). Fluoxetine for acute treatment of depression in children and adolescents: A placebo-controlled, randomized clinical trial. *Journal of the American Academy of Child & Adolescent Psychiatry, 41,* 1205–1215.

Emslie, G. J., Rush, J., Weinberg, W. A., Kowatch, R. A., Hughes, C. W., Carmody, T., & Rintelmann, J. (1997). A double-blind, randomized, placebo-controlled trial of fluoxetine in children and adolescents with depression. *Archives of General Psychiatry, 54,* 1031–1037.

Evans, S. W., Pelham, W. E., & Grudberg, M. V. (1995). The efficacy of notetaking to improve behavior and comprehension of adolescents with attention deficit hyperactivity disorder. *Exceptionality,* 5, 1–17.

Evans, S. W., Pelham, W. E., Smith, B. H., Bukstein, O., Gnagy, E. M., Greiner, A. R., et al. (2001). Dose–response effects of methylphenidate on ecologically valid measures of academic performance and classroom behavior in adolescents with ADHD. *Experimental and Clinical Psychopharmacology*, 9, 163–175.

Fabiano, G. A., & Pelham, W. E. (2002). Evidence-based treatment for mental disorders in children and adolescents. *Current Psychiatry Reports*, *4*, 93–100.

Fabiano, G. A., Pelham, W. E., Burrows-MacLean, L., Gnagy, E. M., Arnold, F., Chacko, A., et al. (in press). The single and combined effects of multiple intensities of behavior modification and medication in a summer treatment program classroom. *School Psychology Review*.

Fabiano, G. A., Pelham, W. E., Coles, E. K., Chronis, A. M., Gnagy, E. M., & O'Connor, B. (2007). *A meta-analysis of behavior modification treatments for ADHD*. Manuscript submitted for publication.

Fava, G. A. (1995). Holding on: Depression, sensitization by antidepressant drugs, and the prodigal experts. *Psychotherapy and Psychosomatics*, *64*, 57–61.

Fava, G. A. (2002). Long-term treatment with antidepressant drugs: The spectacular achievements of propaganda. *Psychotherapy and Psychosomatics*, *71*, 127–132.

Ferdinand, F., & Verhulst, F. C. (1995). Psychopathology from adolescence into young adulthood: An 8-year follow-up study. *American Journal of Psychiatry*, *152*, 1586–1594.

Findling, R. L., Aman, M. G., Eerdekens, M., Derivan, A., Lyons, B., & Risperidone Disruptive Behavior Study Group. (2004). Long-term, open-label study of risperidone in children with severe disruptive behaviors and below-average IQ. *American Journal of Psychiatry*, *161*, 677–684.

Fine, S., Forth, A., Gilbert, M., & Haley, G. (1991). Group therapy for adolescent depressive disorder: A comparison of social skills and therapeutic support. *Journal of the American Academy of Child & Adolescent Psychiatry*, *30*, 79–85.

Fisher, R. L., & Fisher, S. (1996). Antidepressants for children: Is scientific support necessary? *Journal of Nervous and Mental Disease*, *184*, 99–102.

Fleming, J. E., Boyle, M. H., & Offord, D. R. (1993). The outcome of adolescent depression in the Ontario Child Health Study follow-up. *Journal of the American Academy of Child & Adolescent Psychiatry*, *32*, 28–33.

Frankel, F., Myatt, R., Cantwell, D. P., & Feinberg, D. T. (1997). Parent-assisted transfer of children's social skills training: Effects on children with and without attention-deficit hyperactivity disorder. *Journal of the American Academy of Child & Adolescent Psychiatry*, *36*, 1056–1064.

Franklin, L. C., & Johnson, B. (2003). Encopresis. In E. Fletcher-Janzen & C. R. Reynolds (Eds.), *Childhood disorders: Diagnostic desk reference* (pp. 221–222). New York: Wiley.

Frazier, J. A., Biederman, J., Tohen, M., Feldman, P. D., Jacobs, T. G., Toma, V., et al. (2001). A prospective open-label treatment trial of olanzapine monotherapy in children and adolescents with bipolar disorder. *Journal of Child and Adolescent Psychopharmacology*, *11*, 239–250.

Frazier, J. A., Meyer, M. C., Biederman, J., Wozniak, J., Wilens, T. E., Spencer, T. J., et al. (1999). Risperidone treatment for juvenile bipolar disorder: A retrospective chart review. *Journal of the American Academy of Child & Adolescent Psychiatry, 38*, 960–965.

Freeman, R., Fast, D., Burd, L., Kerbeshian, J., Robertson, M., & Sandor, P. (2000). An international perspective on Tourette syndrome: Selected findings from 3500 individuals in 22 countries. *Developmental Medicine & Child Neurology, 42*, 436–447.

Frick, P. J., & Loney, B. R. (1999). Outcomes of children and adolescents with oppositional defiant disorder and conduct disorder. In H. C. Quay & A. E. Hogan (Eds.), *Handbook of disruptive behavior disorders* (pp. 507–524). New York: Kluwer Academic.

Friman, P. C., Osgood, D. W., Shanahan, D., Thompson, R. W., Larzelere, R., & Daly, D. L. (1996). A longitudinal evaluation of prevalent negative beliefs about residential placement for troubled adolescents. *Journal of Abnormal Child Psychology, 24*, 299–324.

Fristad, M. A., Gavazzi, S. M., Centolella, D. M., & Soldano, K. W. (1996). Psychoeducation: A promising intervention strategy for families of children and adolescents with mood disorders. *Contemporary Family Therapy, 18*, 371–383.

Fristad, M. A., Gavazzi, S. M., & Mackinaw-Koons, B. (2003). Family psychoeducation: An adjunctive intervention for children with bipolar disorder. *Biological Psychiatry, 53*, 1000–1008.

Fristad, M. A., Goldberg-Arnold, J. S., & Gavazzi, S. M. (2002). Multifamily psychoeducation groups (MFPG) for families of children with bipolar disorder. *Bipolar Disorders, 4*, 254–262.

Fristad, M. A., Goldberg-Arnold, J. S., & Gavazzi, S. M. (2003). Multifamily psychoeducation groups in the treatment of children with mood disorders. *Journal of Marital and Family Therapy, 29*, 491–504.

Gadow, K. D., Sverd, J., Sprafkin, J., Nolan, E. E., & Ezor, S. N. (1995). Efficacy of methylphenidate for attention-deficit hyperactivity disorder in children with tic disorder. *Archives of General Psychiatry, 52*, 444–445.

Gaffney, G., Perry, P., Lund, B., Bever-Stille, K., Arndt, S., & Kuperman, S. (2002). Risperidone versus clonidine in the treatment of children and adolescents with Tourette's syndrome. *Journal of the American Academy of Child & Adolescent Psychiatry, 41*, 330–336.

Garb, H. N. (2005). Clinical judgment and decision-making. *Annual Review of Clinical Psychology, 1*, 67–89.

Garland, E. J. (2004). Facing the evidence: Antidepressant treatment in children and adolescents. *Canadian Medical Association Journal, 170*, 489–491.

Geist, R., Heinmaa, M., Stephens, D., Davis, R., & Katzman, D. K. (2000). Comparison of family therapy and family group psychoeducation in adolescents with anorexia nervosa. *Canadian Journal of Psychiatry, 45*, 173–178.

Geller, B., Craney, J. L., Bolhofner, K., DelBello, M. P., Williams, M., & Zimerman, B. (2001). One-year recovery and relapse rates of children with a prepubertal and early adolescent bipolar disorder phenotype. *American Journal of Psychiatry, 158*, 303–305.

Geller, B., Craney, J. L., Bolhofner, K., Nickelsburg, M. J., Williams, M., & Zimerman, B. (2002). Two-year prospective follow-up of children with a prepubertal and early adolescent bipolar disorder phenotype. *American Journal of Psychiatry, 159*, 927–933.

Geller, B., Tillman, R., Craney, J. L., & Bolhofner, K. (2004). Four-year prospective outcome and natural history of mania in children with a prepubertal and early adolescent bipolar disorder phenotype. *Archives of General Psychiatry, 61*, 459–467.

Geller, B., Zimerman, B., Williams, M., Bolhofner, K., Craney, J. L., & Delbello, M. P. (2000). Diagnostic characteristics of 93 cases of prepubertal and early adolescent bipolar disorder phenotype by gender, puberty and comorbid attention deficit hyperactivity disorder. *Journal of Child and Adolescent Psychopharmacology, 10*, 157–164.

Geller, D. A., Biederman, J., Faraone, S., Frazier, J., Coffey, B., Kim, G., & Bellordre, C. (2000). Clinical correlates of obsessive compulsive disorder in children and adolescents referred to specialized and non-specialized clinical settings. *Depression and Anxiety, 11*, 163–168.

Geller, D. A., Biederman, J., Stewart, S., Mullin, B., Martin, A., Spencer, T., et al. (2003). Which SSRI? A meta-analysis of pharmacotherapy trials in pediatric obsessive–compulsive disorder. *American Journal of Psychiatry, 160*, 1919–1928.

Geller, D. A., Hoog, S. L., Heiligenstein, J. H., Ricardi, R. K., Tamura, R., Kluszynski, S., & Jacobson, J. G. (2001). The fluoxetine pediatric OCD study team, U.S. fluoxetine treatment for obsessive–compulsive disorder in children and adolescents: A placebo-controlled clinical trial. *Journal of the American Academy of Child & Adolescent Psychiatry, 40*, 773–779.

Gerardin, P., Cohen, D., Mazet, P., & Flament, M. F. (2002). Drug treatment of conduct disorder in young people. *European Neuropsychopharmacology, 12*, 361–370.

Gilbert, D. (2006). Treatment of children and adolescents with tics and Tourette syndrome. *Journal of Child Neurology, 21*, 690–700.

Gilbert, D., Batterson, J., Sethuraman, G., & Sallee, F. (2004). Tic reduction with risperidone versus pimozide in a randomized, double-blind, crossover trial. *Journal of the American Academy of Child & Adolescent Psychiatry, 43*, 206–214.

Gittelman, R., Abikoff, H., Pollack, E., Klein, D. F., Katz, S., & Mattes, J. (1980). A controlled trial of behavior modification and methylphenidate in hyperactive children. In C. K. Whalen & B. Henker (Eds.), *Hyperactive children: The social ecology of identification and treatment* (pp. 221–243). New York: Academic Press.

Gittelman-Klein, R., & Klein, D. F. (1973). Controlled imipramine treatment of school phobia. *Archives of General Psychiatry, 25*, 199–215.

GlaxoSmithKline. (n.d.). *Use of Paxil or Paxil CR in pediatric patients*. Retrieved May 7, 2007, from http://www.gsk.com/media/paroxetine/letter.pdf

Goldberg-Arnold, J. S., Fristad, M. A., & Gavazzi, S. M. (1999). Family psychoeducation: Giving caregivers what they want and need. *Family Relations*, *48*, 411–417.

Goode, E. (2004, February 3). Stronger warning is urged on antidepressants for teenagers. *New York Times*, p. A12.

Gordon, C. T., State, R. C., Nelson, J. E., Hamburger, S. D., & Rapoport, J. L. (1993). A double-blind comparison of clomipramine, desipramine, and placebo in the treatment of autistic disorder. *Archives of General Psychiatry*, *50*, 441–447.

Gowers, S., & Bryant-Waugh, R. (2004). Management of child and adolescent eating disorders: The current evidence base and future directions. *Journal of Child Psychology and Psychiatry*, *45*, 63–83.

Graae, F., Milner, J., Rizzoto, L., & Klein, R. G. (1994). Clonazepam in childhood anxiety disorders. *Journal of the American Academy of Child & Adolescent Psychiatry*, *33*, 372–376.

Greenhill, L. L., & Ford, R. E. (2006). Childhood attention-deficit hyperactivity disorder: Psychopharmacological treatments. In P. E. Nathan & J. M. Gorman (Eds.), *A guide to treatments that work* (pp. 25–56). New York: Oxford University Press.

Greenhill, L. L., Kollins, S., Abikoff, H., McCracken, J., Riddle, M., Swanson, J., et al. (2006). Efficacy and safety of immediate-release methylphenidate treatment for preschoolers with ADHD. *Journal of the American Academy of Child & Adolescent Psychiatry*, *45*, 1284–1293.

Greenhill, L. L., Swanson, J. M., Vitiello, B., Davies, M., Clevenger, W., Wu, M., et al. (2001). Impairment and deportment responses to different methylphenidate doses in children with ADHD: The MTA titration trial. *Journal of the American Academy of Child & Adolescent Psychiatry*, *40*, 180–187.

Greenhill, L. L., Vitiello, B., Abikoff, H., Levine, J., March, J. S., Riddle, M. A., et al. (2003). Developing methodologies for monitoring long-term safety of psychotropic medications in children: Report on the NIMH Conference, Sept. 25, 2000. *Journal of the American Academy of Child & Adolescent Psychiatry*, *42*, 651–655.

Grunbaum, J. A., Kann, L., Kinchen, S., Ross, J., Hawkins, J., Lowry, R., et al. (2004). Youth Risk Behavior Surveillance—United States, 2003. *MMWR Surveillance Summary*, *53*(2), 1–96.

Guevara, J., Lozano, P., Wickizer, T., Mell, L., & Gephart, H. (2002). Psychotropic medication use in a population of children who have attention-deficit/hyperactivity disorder. *Pediatrics*, *109*, 733–739.

Gurley, D., Cohen, P., Pine, D. S., & Brook, J. (1996). Discriminating depression and anxiety in youth: A role for diagnostic criteria. *Journal of Affective Disorders*, *39*, 191–200.

Gutkind, D., Ventura, J., Barr, C., Shaner, A., Green, M., & Mintz, J. (2001). Factors affecting reliability and confidence of *DSM–III–R* psychosis-related diagnosis. *Psychiatry Research*, *101*, 269–275.

Guy, W. (1976). *ECDEU assessment manual for psychopharmacology* (Rev.; DHEW publication no. [ADM] 76-338). Rockville, MD: National Institute of Mental Health.

Halbreich, U., Shen, J., & Panaro, V. (1996). Are chronic psychiatric patients at increased risk for developing breast cancer? *American Journal of Psychiatry, 153*, 559–560.

Hall, L. H., & Robertson, M. H. (1998). Undergraduate ratings of the acceptability of single and combined treatments for depression: A comparative analysis. *Professional Psychology: Research and Practice, 29*, 269–272.

Hammad, T. A., Laughren, T., & Racoosin, J. (2006). Suicidality in pediatric patients treated with antidepressant drugs. *Archives of General Psychiatry, 63*, 332–339.

Hankin, B. L., Abramson, L. Y., Moffitt, T. E., Silva, P. A., McGee, R., & Angell, K. E. (1998). Development of depression from preadolescence to young adulthood: Emerging gender differences in a 10-year longitudinal study. *Journal of Abnormal Psychology, 107*, 128–140.

Harrigan, S. M., McGorry, P. D., & Hrstev, H. (2003). Does treatment delay in first-episode psychosis really matter? *Psychological Medicine, 33*, 97–110.

Harrington, R., Kerfoot, M., Dyer, E., McNiven, F., Gill, J., Harrington, V., et al. (1998). Randomized trial of a home-based family intervention of children who have deliberately poisoned themselves. *Journal of the American Academy of Child & Adolescent Psychiatry, 37*, 512–518.

Harris, S. L. (1995). Autism. In M. Hersen & R. L. Ammerman (Eds.), *Advanced abnormal child psychology* (pp. 305–317). Hillsdale, NJ: Erlbaum.

Hartman, R. R., Stage, S. A., & Webster-Stratton, C. (2003). A growth curve analysis of parent training outcomes: Examining the influence of child risk factors (inattention, impulsivity, and hyperactivity problems), parental and family risk factors. *Journal of Child Psychology and Psychiatry and Allied Disciplines, 44*, 388–398.

Hay, P. J., Bacaltchuk, J., & Stefano, S. (2004). Psychotherapy for bulimia nervosa and binging (CD000562). *Cochrane Database of Systematic Reviews*. Available at http://www.cochrane.org/reviews/en/ab000562.html

Hazell, P., O'Connell, D., Heathcote, D., Robertson, J., & Henry, D. (1995). Efficacy of tricyclic drugs in treating child and adolescent depression: A meta-analysis. *British Medical Journal, 310*, 897–901.

Hazell, P. L., & Stuart, J. E. (2003). A randomized controlled trial of clonidine added to psychostimulant medication for hyperactive and aggressive children. *Journal of the American Academy of Child & Adolescent Psychiatry, 42*, 886–894.

Healy, D. (2003). Lines of evidence on the risks of suicide with selective serotonin reuptake inhibitors. *Psychotherapy and Psychosomatics, 72*, 71–79.

Henggeler, S. W., Schoenwald, S. K., Rowland, M. D., & Cunningham, P. B. (2002). *Serious emotional disturbance in children and adolescents: Multisystemic therapy*. New York: Guilford.

Henry, C. (2002). Lithium side-effects and predictors of hypothyroidism in patients with bipolar disorder: Sex differences. *Journal of Psychiatry & Neuroscience, 27,* 104–107.

Hinshaw, S., March, J., Abikoff, H., Arnold, L. E., Cantwell, D. P., Conners, C. K., et al. (1997). Comprehensive assessment of childhood ADHD in the context of a multisite, multimodal clinical trial. *Journal of Attention Disorders, 1,* 217–234.

Hirshberg, L. M., Chiu, S., & Frazier, J. A. (2005). Emerging brain-based interventions for children and adolescents: Overview and clinical perspective. *Child and Adolescent Psychiatric Clinics of North America, 14,* 1–19.

Hollander, E., Phillips, A., Chaplin, W., Zagursky, K., Novotny, S., Wasserman, S., & Iyengar, R. (2005). A placebo controlled crossover trial of liquid fluoxetine on repetitive behaviors in childhood and adolescent autism. *Neuropsychopharmacology, 30,* 582–599.

Hollon, S. D., DeRubeis, R. J., Shelton, R. C., Amsterdam, J. D., Salomon, R. M., O'Reardon, J. P., et al. (2005). Prevention of relapse following cognitive therapy vs. medications in moderate to severe depression. *Archives of General Psychiatry, 62,* 417–422.

Hook, C. L., & DuPaul, G. J. (1999). Parent tutoring for students with attention-deficit/hyperactivity disorder: Effects on reading performance at home and school. *School Psychology Review, 28,* 60–75.

Houts, A. C., Berman, J. S., & Abramson, H. A. (1994). The effectiveness of psychological and pharmacological treatments for nocturnal enuresis. *Journal of Consulting and Clinical Psychology, 62,* 737–745.

Huey, S. J., Jr., Henggeler, S. W., Rowland, M. D., Halliday-Boykins, C. A., Cunningham, P. B., Pickrel, S. G., & Edwards, J. (2004). Multisystemic therapy effects on attempted suicide by youths presenting psychiatric emergencies. *Journal of the American Academy of Child & Adolescent Psychiatry, 43,* 183–190.

Hunsley, J. (2003). Cost-effectiveness and medical cost offset considerations in psychological service provision. *Canadian Psychology, 44,* 61–73.

Hyman, S. E. (2000). The millennium of mind, brain, and behavior. *Archives of General Psychiatry, 57,* 88–89.

Ialongo, N., Edelsohn, G., Werthamer-Larsson, L., Crockett, L., & Kellam, S. (1994). The significance of self-reported anxious symptoms in first-grade children. *Journal of Abnormal Child Psychology, 22,* 441–455.

Institute of Medicine. (2001). *Crossing the quality chasm: A new health system for the 21st century.* Washington, DC: National Academy Press.

Jager, B., Liedtke, R., Lamprecht, F., & Freyberger, H. (2004). Social and health adjustment of bulimic women 7–9 years following therapy. *Acta Psychiatrica Scandinavica, 110,* 138–145.

Jenike, M. (1990). Psychotherapy of obsessive compulsive personality disorder. In M. Jenike, L. Baer, & W. Minichello (Eds.), *Obsessive–compulsive disorders: Theory and management* (pp. 295–305). Chicago: Year Book Medical.

Jensen, P. S., Bhatara, V. S., Vitiello, B., Hoagwood, K., Feil, M., & Burke, L. B. (1999). Psychoactive medication prescribing practices for U.S. children: Gaps between research and clinical practice. *Journal of the American Academy of Child & Adolescent Psychiatry, 38*, 557–565.

Jensen, P. S., Hinshaw, S. P., Kraemer, H. C., Lenora, N., Newcorn, J. H., Abikoff, H. B., et al. (2001). ADHD comorbidity findings from the MTA study: Comparing comorbid subgroups. *Journal of the American Academy of Child & Adolescent Psychiatry, 40*, 147–158.

Jensen, P. S., Weersing, R., Hoagwood, K. E., & Goldman, E. (2005). What is the evidence for evidence-based treatments? A hard look at our soft underbelly. *Mental Health Services Research, 7*, 53–74.

Johnson, S. B. (1980). Enuresis. In R. Daitzman (Ed.), *Clinical behavior therapy and behavior modification* (pp. 81–142). New York: Garland.

Johnson, W. G., Tsoh, J. Y., & Varnado, P. J. (1996). Eating disorders: Efficacy of pharmacological and psychological interventions. *Clinical Psychology Review, 16*, 457–478.

Jorm, A. F. (2000). Mental health literacy: Public knowledge and beliefs about mental disorders. *British Journal of Psychiatry, 177*, 396–401.

Joukamaa, M., Heliovaara, M., Knekt, P., Aromaa, A., Raitasalo, R., & Lehtinen, V. (2006). Schizophrenia, neuroleptic medication and mortality. *British Journal of Psychiatry, 188*, 122–127.

Jureidini, J. N., Doecke, C. J., Mansfield, P. R., Haby, M. M., Menkes, D. B., & Tonkin, A. L. (2004). Efficacy and safety of antidepressants for children and adolescents. *British Medical Journal, 328*, 879–883.

Kafantaris, V., Coletti, D. J., Dicker, R., Padula, G., & Kane, J. M. (2001). Adjunctive antipsychotic treatment of adolescents with bipolar psychosis. *Journal of the American Academy of Child & Adolescent Psychiatry, 40*, 1448–1456.

Kafantaris, V., Coletti, D. J., Dicker, R., Padula, G., & Kane, J. M. (2003). Lithium treatment of acute mania in adolescents: A large open trial. *Journal of the American Academy of Child & Adolescent Psychiatry, 42*, 1038–1045.

Kahn, J. S., Kehle, T. J., Jenson, W. R., & Clark, E. (1990). Comparison of cognitive–behavioral, relaxation and self-modeling interventions for depression among middle-school students. *School Psychology Review, 19*, 196–211.

Kahng, S. W., Iwata, B. A., & Lewin, A. B. (2002). The impact of functional assessment on the treatment of self-injurious behavior. In S. R. Shroeder, M. L. Oster-Granite, & T. Travis (Eds.), *Self-injurious behavior: Gene–brain–behavior relationships* (pp. 119–131). Washington, DC: American Psychological Association.

Kann, R. T., & Hanna, F. J. (2000). Disruptive behavior disorders in children and adolescents: How do girls differ from boys? *Journal of Counseling and Development, 78*, 267–274.

Kaslow, N. J., & Thompson, M. P. (1998). Applying the criteria for empirically supported treatments to studies of psychosocial interventions for child and adolescent depression. *Journal of Clinical Child Psychology, 27*, 146–155.

Katz, L. Y., Cox, B. J., Gunasekara, S., & Miller, A. L. (2004). Feasibility of dialectical behavior therapy for suicidal adolescent inpatients. *Journal of the American Academy of Child & Adolescent Psychiatry, 43*, 276–282.

Kaye, W. H., Bulik, C. M., Thornton, L., Barbarich, N., Masters, K., & The Price Foundation Collaborative Group. (2004). Comorbidity of anxiety disorders with anorexia and bulimia nervosa. *American Journal of Psychiatry, 161*, 2215–2221.

Kaye, W. H., Nagata, T., Weltzin, T. E., Hsu, G., Sokol, M. S., Conaha, C. M., et al. (2001). Double-blind placebo controlled administration of fluoxetine in restricting- and restricting-purging-type anorexia nervosa. *Biological Psychiatry, 49*, 644–652.

Kazdin, A. E. (2000). Treatments for aggressive and antisocial children. *Child and Adolescent Psychiatry Clinics of North America, 9*, 841–858.

Kazdin, A. E., Siegel, T. C., & Bass, D. (1992). Cognitive problem-solving skills training and parent management training in the treatment of antisocial behavior in children. *Journal of Consulting and Clinical Psychology, 60*, 737–747.

Keenan, K., Loeber, R., & Green, S. (1999). Conduct disorder in girls: A review of the literature. *Clinical Child and Family Psychology Review, 2*, 3–19.

Keller, M., Ryan, N., Strober, M., Klein, R., Kutcher, S., Birmaher, B., et al. (2001). Efficacy of paroxetine in the treatment of adolescent major depression: A randomized, controlled trial. *Journal of the American Academy of Child & Adolescent Psychiatry, 40*, 762–772.

Kendall, P. C. (1994). Treating anxiety disorders in children: Results of a randomized clinical trial. *Journal of Consulting and Clinical Psychology, 62*, 100–110.

Kendall, P. C., & Brady, E. U. (1995). Comorbidity in the anxiety disorders of childhood: Implications for validity and clinical significance. In K. D. Craig & K. S. Dobson (Eds.), *Anxiety and depression in adults and children* (pp. 3–36). Thousand Oaks, CA: Sage.

Kendall, P. C., Flannery-Schroeder, E., Panichelli-Mindel, S. M., Southam-Gerow, M., Henin, A., & Warman, M. (1997). Therapy for youths with anxiety disorders: A second randomized clinical trial. *Journal of Consulting and Clinical Psychology, 65*, 366–380.

Kendall, P. C., Safford, S. M., Flannery-Schroeder, E., & Webb, A. (2004). Child anxiety treatment: Outcomes and impact on substance use and depression 7.5 years later. *Journal of Consulting and Clinical Psychology, 72*, 276–287.

Kendall, P. C., & Southam-Gerow, M. A. (1996). Long-term follow-up of a cognitive–behavioral therapy for anxiety-disordered youth. *Journal of Consulting and Clinical Psychology, 64*, 724–730.

Kendall, T., Pilling, S., & Whittington, C. J. (2005). Are the SSRIs and atypical antidepressants safe and effective for children and adolescents? *Current Opinions in Psychiatry, 18*, 21–25.

Kessler, R. C., Avenevoli, S., & Merikangas, K. R. (2001). Mood disorders in children and adolescents: An epidemiological perspective. *Biological Psychiatry, 49*, 1002–1014.

Kessler, R. C., McGonagle, K. A., Zhao, S., Nelson, C. B., Hughes, M., Eshleman, S., et al. (1994). Lifetime and 12-month prevalence of *DSM–III–R* psychiatric disorders in the United States: Results from the National Comorbidity Study. *Archives of General Psychiatry, 51,* 8–19.

King, C. A., Hovey, J. D., Brand, E., Wilson, R., & Ghaziuddin, N. (1997). Suicidal adolescents after hospitalization: Parent and family impacts on treatment follow-through. *Journal of the American Academy of Child & Adolescent Psychiatry, 35,* 743–751.

King, C. A., Kramer, A., Preuss, L., Kerr, D. C. R., Weisse, L., & Venkataraman, S. (2006). Youth-nominated support team for suicidal adolescents (Version 1): A randomized controlled trial. *Journal of Consulting and Clinical Psychology, 74,* 199–206.

King, N. J., Tonge, B. J., Mullen, P., Myerson, N., Heyne, D., Rollings, S., et al. (2000). Treating sexually abused children with posttraumatic stress symptoms: A randomized clinical trial. *Journal of the American Academy of Child & Adolescent Psychiatry, 39,* 1347–1355.

King, R. A., Riddle, M. A., Chappell, P. B., Hardin, M. T., Anderson, G. M., Lombroso, P., & Scahill, L. (1991). Emergence of self-destructive phenomena in children and adolescents during fluoxetine treatment. *Journal of the American Academy of Child & Adolescent Psychiatry, 30,* 179–186.

Klaus, N., & Fristad, M. A. (in press). Mood disorders. In M. L. Wolraich, P. H., Dworkin, D. D. Drotar, & E. Perrin (Eds.), *Developmental and behavioral pediatrics.* Philadelphia: Elsevier.

Klaus, N., Fristad, M. A., Malkin, C., & Koons, B. M. (2005, November). *Psychosocial family treatment for a nine-year-old with schizoaffective disorder.* Poster presented at the 39th Annual Association for Behavioral and Cognitive Therapy, Washington, DC.

Klein, R. G., & Abikoff, H. (1997). Behavior therapy and methylphenidate in the treatment of children with ADHD. *Journal of Attention Disorders, 2,* 89–114.

Klein, R. G., Abikoff, H., Ganeles, D., Seese, L. M., & Pollack, S. (1997). Clinical efficacy of methylphenidate in conduct disorder with and without attention deficit hyperactivity disorder. *Archives of General Psychiatry, 54,* 1073–1080.

Klein, R. G., Koplewicz, H., & Kanner, A. (1992). Imipramine treatment of children with separation anxiety disorder. *Journal of the American Academy of Child & Adolescent Psychiatry, 31,* 21–28.

Klerman, G. L., Weissman, M. M., Rounsaville, B. J., & Chevron, E. S. (1984). *Interpersonal psychotherapy of depression.* New York: Basic Books.

Klin, A., Lang, J., Cicchetti, D., & Volkmar, F. (2001). Autistic disorder: Results of the *DSM–IV* autism field trial. *Journal of Developmental and Autism Disorders, 330,* 163–167.

Kobe, F. H., & Mulick, J. A. (1995). Mental retardation. In R. T. Ammerman & M. Hersen (Eds.), *Handbook of child behavior therapy in the psychiatric setting* (pp. 153–180). New York: Wiley.

Koegel, R. L., & Koegel, L. K. (1995). *Teaching children with autism: Strategies for initiating positive interactions and improving learning opportunities*. Baltimore: Paul H. Brookes.

Koegel, R. L., Koegel, L. K., & Brookman, L. I. (2003). Empirically supported pivotal response interventions for children with autism. In A. E. Kazdin & J. R. Weisz (Eds.), *Evidence-based psychotherapies for children and adolescents* (pp. 341–347). New York: Guilford Press.

Kolko, D. J., Bukstein, O. G., & Barron, J. (1999). Methylphenidate and behavior modification in children with ADHD and comorbid ODD or CD: Main and incremental effects across settings. *Journal of the American Academy of Child & Adolescent Psychiatry, 38*, 578–586.

Kovacs, M. (1996). Presentation and course of major depressive disorder during childhood and later years of the lifespan. *Journal of the American Academy of Child & Adolescent Psychiatry, 35*, 705–715.

Kovacs, M. (2003). *Children's Depression Inventory—Revised.* North Tonawanda, NY: Multi-Health Systems.

Kovacs, M., Goldston, D., & Gatsonis, C. (1993). Suicidal behaviors and childhood-onset depressive disorders: A longitudinal investigation. *Journal of the American Academy of Child & Adolescent Psychiatry, 32*, 8–20.

Kovacs, M., Obrosky, S., Gatsonis, C., & Richards, C. (1997). First-episode major depressive and dysthymic disorder in childhood: Clinical and sociodemographic factors in recovery. *Journal of the American Academy of Child & Adolescent Psychiatry, 36*, 777–784.

Kowatch, R. A., & Fristad, M. A. (2006). Pediatric bipolar disorders. In R. T. Ammerman (Ed.), M. Hersen, & J. C. Thomas (Chief Eds.), *Comprehensive handbook of personality and psychopathology: Vol. III. Child psychopathology* (pp. 217–232). New York: Wiley.

Kowatch, R. A., Fristad, M. A., Birmaher, B., Wagner, K. D., Findling, R. L., Hellander, M., & Child Psychiatric Workgroup on Bipolar Disorder. (2005). Treatment guidelines for children and adolescents with bipolar disorder. *Journal of the American Academy of Child & Adolescent Psychiatry, 44*, 213–235.

Kowatch, R. A., Suppes, T., Carmody, T. J., Bucci, J. P., Hume, J. H., Kromelis, M., et al. (2000). Effect size of lithium, divalproex sodium, and carbamazepine in children and adolescents with bipolar disorder. *Journal of the American Academy of Child & Adolescent Psychiatry, 39*, 713–720.

Kowatch, R. A., Suppes, T., Gilfillan, S. K., Fuentes, R. M., Granneman, B. D., & Emslie, G. J. (1995). Clozapine treatment of children and adolescents with bipolar disorder and schizophrenia: A clinical case series. *Journal of Child and Adolescent Psychopharmacology, 5*, 241–253.

Kozak, M. J., & Foa, E. B. (1997). *Mastery of obsessive–compulsive disorder: A cognitive–behavioral approach* (Therapist guide). San Antonio, TX: Psychological Corporation.

Kuehn, B. M. (2007). Cognitive–behavioral therapy shows promise for children with mental illness. *Journal of the American Medical Association, 297*, 453–455.

Kurlan, R., Goetz, C. G., McDermott, M. P., Plumb, S., Singer, H., Dure, L., et al. (2002). Treatment of ADHD in children with tics: A randomized controlled trial. *Neurology, 58,* 527–536.

Kusumaker, V., & Yatham, L. N. (1997). Lamotrigine treatment of rapidly cycling bipolar disorder. *American Journal of Psychiatry, 154,* 1171–1172.

La Greca, A. M., & Bearman, K. J. (2003). Adherence to pediatric regimens. In M. C. Roberts (Ed.), *Handbook of pediatric psychology* (3rd ed.). New York: Guilford Press.

Lasser, K. E., Allen, P. D., Woolhandler, S. J., Himmelstein, D. U., Wolfe, S. M., & Bor, D. H. (2002). Timing of new black box warnings and withdrawals for prescription medications. *Journal of the American Medical Association, 287,* 2215–2220.

Last, C. G., Hansen, C., & Franco, N. (1998). Cognitive–behavioral treatment of social phobia. *Journal of the American Academy of Child & Adolescent Psychiatry, 37,* 404–411.

Last, C. G., Hersen, M., Kazdin, A., Orvaschel, H., & Perrin, S. (1991). Anxiety disorders in children and their families. *Archives of General Psychiatry, 48,* 928–934.

Leckman, J., King, R., Scahill, L., Findley, D., Ort, S., & Cohen, D. (1999). Yale approach to assessment and treatment. In J. F. Leckman & D. J. Cohen (Eds.), *Tourette's syndrome—Tics, obsessions, compulsions: Developmental psychopathology and clinical care* (pp. 285–309). Hoboken, NJ: Wiley.

Leckman, J., Zhang, H., Vitale, A., Lahnin, F., Lynch, K., Bondi, C., et al. (1998). Course of tic severity in Tourette syndrome: The first two decades. *Pediatrics, 102,* 14–19.

Lenior, M. E., Dingemans, P., Linszen, D. H., de Haan, L., & Schene, A. H. (2001). Social functioning and the course of early-onset schizophrenia: Five-year follow-up of a psychosocial intervention. *British Journal of Psychiatry, 179,* 53–58.

Leonard, H., Ale, C., Freeman, J., Garcia, A., & Nigg, J. (2005). Obsessive–compulsive disorder. *Child and Adolescent Psychiatric Clinics of North America, 14,* 727–743.

Leucht, S., Pitschel-Walz, G., Abraham, D., & Kissling, W. (1999). Efficacy and extrapyramidal side-effects of the new antipsychotics olanzapine, quetiapine, risperidone, and sertindole compared to conventional antipsychotics and placebo. A meta-analysis of randomized controlled trials. *Schizophrenia Research, 35,* 51–68.

Levinsky, N. G. (2002). Nonfinancial conflicts of interest in research. *New England Journal of Medicine, 347,* 759–761.

Lewinsohn, P. M., & Clarke, G. N. (1984). Group treatment of depressed individuals: The "coping with depression" course. *Advances in Behavior Research and Therapy, 6,* 99–114.

Lewinsohn, P. M., Clarke, G. N., Hops, H., & Andrews, J. (1990). Cognitive–behavioral treatment of depressed adolescents. *Behavior Therapy, 21,* 385–401.

Lewinsohn, P. M., Clarke, G. N., Seeley, J. R., & Rohde, P. (1994). Major depression in community adolescents: Age at onset, episode duration, and time to recurrence. *Journal of the American Academy of Child & Adolescent Psychiatry, 33,* 809–818.

Lewinsohn, P. M., Hops, H., Roberts, R. E., Seeley, J. R., & Andrews, J. A. (1993). Adolescent psychopathology: I. Prevalence and incidence of depression and other *DSM–III–R* disorders in high school students. *Journal of Abnormal Psychology, 103,* 133–144.

Lewinsohn, P. M., Seeley, J. R., & Klein, D. N. (1995). Bipolar disorder in a community sample of older adolescents: Prevalence, phenomenology, comorbidity, and course. *Journal of the American Academy of Child & Adolescent Psychiatry, 34,* 454–463.

Liddle, B., & Spence, S. H. (1990). Cognitive–behavioral therapy with depressed primary school children: A cautionary note. *Behavioral Psychotherapy, 18,* 85–102.

Lieberman, J. A., Stroup, T. S., McEvoy, J. P., Swartz, M. S., Rosenheck, R. A., Perkins, D. O., et al. (2005). Clinical Antipsychotic Trials of Intervention Effectiveness (CATIE) investigators. *New England Journal of Medicine, 353,* 1209–1223.

Liebowitz, M., Turner, S., Piacentini, J., Beidel, D., Clarvit, S., Davies, S., et al. (2002). Fluoxetine in children and adolescents with OCD: A placebo-controlled trial. *Journal of the American Academy of Child & Adolescent Psychiatry, 41,* 1431–1438.

Lin, K. M., Poland, R. E., & Nakasaki, G. (1993). *Psychopharmacology and psychobiology of ethnicity.* Washington, DC: American Psychiatric Press.

Linehan, M. M., Armstrong, H. E., Suarez, A., Allmon, D., & Heard, H. L. (1991). Cognitive–behavioral treatment of chronically parasuicidal borderline patients. *Archives of General Psychiatry, 48,* 1060–1064.

Linehan, M. M., Heard, H. L., & Armstrong, H. E. (1993). Naturalistic follow-up of a behavioral treatment for chronically parasuicidal borderline patients. *Archives of General Psychiatry, 50,* 971–974.

Lipkin, P. H., Cozen, M. A., Thompson, R. E., & Mostofsky, S. H. (2005). Stimulant dosage and age, race, and insurance type in a sample of children with attention-deficit/hyperactivity disorder. *Journal of Child and Adolescent Psychopharmacology, 15,* 240–248.

Lochman, J. E., & Wells, K. C. (2004). The Coping Power program for preadolescent aggressive boys and their parents: Outcome effects at the 1-year follow-up. *Journal of Consulting and Clinical Psychology, 72,* 571–578.

Loening-Baucke, V. I. (1989). Factors determining outcome in children with chronic constipation and faecal soiling. *Gut, 30,* 999–1006.

Lord, C., Wagner, A., Rogers, S., Szatmari, P., Aman, M., Charman, T., et al. (2005). Challenges in evaluating psychosocial interventions for autistic spectrum disorders. *Journal of Autism Developmental Disorders, 35,* 695–708.

Lovaas, O. I. (1987). Behavioral treatment and normal educational and intellectual functioning in young autistic children. *Journal of Consulting and Clinical Psychology, 55,* 3–9.

Lovaas, O. I., & Smith, T. (2003). Early and intensive behavioral intervention in autism. In A. E. Kazdin & J. R. Weisz (Eds.), *Evidence-based psychotherapies for children and adolescents* (pp. 325–340). New York: Guilford Press.

Luby, E. D., & Singareddy, R. K. (2003). Long-term therapy with lithium in a private practice clinic: A naturalistic study. *Bipolar Disorders, 5,* 62–68.

Lundahl, B., Risser, H. J., & Lovejoy, C. M. (2006). A meta-analysis of parent training: Moderators and follow-up effects. *Clinical Psychology Review, 26,* 86–104.

Malone, R. P., Delaney, M. A., Leubbert, J. F., Cater, J., & Campbell, M. (2000). A double-blind, placebo-controlled study of lithium in hospitalized aggressive children and adolescents with conduct disorder. *Archives of General Psychiatry, 57,* 649–654.

March, J. S., & Curry, J. (1998). Predicting the outcome of treatment. *Journal of Abnormal Child Psychology, 26,* 39–51.

March, J. S., Frances, A., Carpenter, D., & Kahn, D. (1997). Expert consensus guidelines: Treatment of obsessive–compulsive disorder. *Journal of Clinical Psychiatry, 58,* 1–72.

March, J. S., Leonard, H., & Swedo, S. (1995). Obsessive–compulsive disorder. In J. S. March (Ed.), *Anxiety disorders in children and adolescents* (pp. 251–275). New York: Guilford Press.

March, J. S., & Mulle, K. (1998). *OCD in children and adolescents: A cognitive–behavioral treatment manual.* New York: Guilford Press.

March, J. S., & Ollendick, T. H. (2004). Integrated psychosocial and pharmacological treatment. In T. H. Ollendick & J. S. March (Eds.), *Phobic and anxiety disorders in children and adolescents: A clinician's guide to effective psychosocial and pharmacological interventions* (pp. 141–172). New York: Oxford University Press.

Marttunen, M. J., Aro, H. M., Henriksson, M. M., & Lonnqvist, J. K. (1991). Mental disorders in adolescent suicide: *DSM–III–R* Axes I and II diagnoses in suicides among 13- to 19-year-olds in Finland. *Archives of General Psychiatry, 48,* 834–839.

Mash, E. J., & Hunsley, J. (Eds.). (2005). Evidence-based assessment of child and adolescent disorders: Issues and challenges [Special section]. *Journal of Clinical Child and Adolescent Psychology, 34,* 362–558.

Maughan, D. R., Christiansen, E., Jenson, W. R., Olympia, D., & Clark, E. (2005). Behavioral parent training as a treatment for externalizing behaviors and disruptive behavior disorders: A meta-analysis. *School Psychology Review, 34,* 267–286.

McClellan, J., Werry, J. S., & Work Group on Quality Issues. (2001). Practice parameter for the assessment and treatment of children and adolescents with schizophrenia. *Journal of the American Academy of Child & Adolescent Psychiatry, 40*(Suppl. 7), 4S–23S.

McCracken, J., Sallee, F., Leonard, H., Allen, A. J., Budman, C. L., Geller, D., et al. (2003, October). *Improvement of ADHD by atomoxetine in children with tic disorders*. Paper presented at the annual meeting of the American Academy of Child & Adolescent Psychiatry, Miami, FL.

McDougle, C. J., Scahill, L., Aman, M. G., McCracken, J. T., Tierney, E., Davies, M., et al. (2005). Risperidone for the core symptom domains of autism: Results from the RUPP Autism Network Study. *American Journal of Psychiatry, 162*, 1142–1148.

McGorry, P. D., Yung, A. R., Phillips, L. J., Yuen, H. P., Francey, S. F., Cosgrave, E. M., et al. (2002). Randomized controlled trial of interventions designed to reduce the risk of progression to first-episode psychosis in a clinical sample with subthreshold symptoms. *Archives of General Psychiatry, 59*, 921–928.

McGrath, M. L., Mellon, M. W., & Murphy, L. (2000). Empirically supported treatments in pediatric psychology: Constipation and encopresis. *Journal of Pediatric Psychology, 25*, 225–254.

McIntosh, V. V., Jordan, J., Carter, F. A., Luty, S. E., McKenzie, J. M., Bulik, C. M., et al. (2005). Three psychotherapies for anorexia nervosa: A randomized, controlled trial. *American Journal of Psychiatry, 162*, 741–747.

Mehler, C., Wewetzer, C., Schulze, W., Wamke, A., Theisen, F., & Dittmann, R.W. (2001). Olanzapine in children and adolescents with chronic anorexia nervosa. A study of five cases. *European Child and Adolescent Psychiatry, 10*, 151–157.

Meighen, K. G., Shelton, H. M., & McDougle, C. J. (2004). Case report: Ziprasidone treatment of two adolescents with psychosis. *Journal of Child and Adolescent Psychopharmacology, 14*, 137–142.

Mellon, M. W., & Houts, A. C. (1998). Home-based treatment for primary enuresis. In J. Briesmeister & C. E. Schaefer (Eds.), *Handbook of parent training: Parents as co-therapists for children's behavior problems* (2nd ed., pp. 384–417). New York: Wiley.

Mellon, M. W., & McGrath, M. L. (2000). Empirically supported treatments in pediatric psychology: Nocturnal enuresis. *Journal of Pediatric Psychology, 25*, 193–214.

Meyer, V. (1966). Modification of expectations in cases with obsessive rituals. *Behavioral Research and Therapy, 4*, 270–280.

Michael, K. D., & Crowley, S. L. (2002). How effective are treatments for children and adolescent depression? A meta-analytic review. *Clinical Psychology Review, 22*, 247–269.

Michelson, D., Faries, D., Wernicke, J., Kelsey, D., Kendrick, K., Sallee, F. R., & Spencer, T. (2001). Atomoxetine in the treatment of children and adolescents with attention-deficit/hyperactivity disorder: A randomized, placebo-controlled, dose-response study. *Pediatrics, 108*, E83.

Miklowitz, D. J., George, E. L., Axelson, D. A., Kim, E. Y., Birmaher, B., Schneck, C., et al. (2004). Family-focused treatment for adolescents with bipolar disorder. *Journal of Affective Disorders, 82*(Suppl. 1), 113–128.

Moffatt, M. E. (1997). Nocturnal enuresis: A review of the efficacy of treatments and practical advice for clinicians. *Developmental and Behavioral Pediatrics, 18*, 49–56.

Moffatt, M. E., Harlos, S., Kirshen, A. J., & Burd, L. (1993). Desmopressin acetate and nocturnal enuresis: How much do we know? *Pediatrics, 92*, 420–424.

Moffitt, T. E., Caspi, A., Dickson, N., Silva, P., & Stanton, W. (1996). Childhood-onset versus adolescent-onset antisocial conduct problems in males: Natural history from ages 3 to 18 years. *Development and Psychopathology, 8*, 399–424.

Moher, D., Schulz, K. F., & Altman, D. (2001). The CONSORT statement: Revised recommendations for improving the quality of reports of parallel-group randomized trials. *Journal of the American Medical Association, 285*, 1987–1991.

Moorman, P. G., Grubber, J. M., Millikan, R. C., & Newman, B. (2003). Antidepressant medications and their association with invasive breast cancer and carcinoma in situ of the breast. *Epidemiology, 14*, 307– 314.

Mrug, S., Hoza, B., & Gerdes, A. C. (2001). Children with attention-deficit/hyperactivity disorder: Peer relationships and peer-oriented interventions. In D. W. Nangle & C. A. Erdley (Eds.), *The role of friendship in psychological adjustment: New directions for child and adolescent development* (pp. 51–77). San Francisco: Jossey-Bass.

Mueser, K. T., & McGurk, S. R. (2004). Schizophrenia. *The Lancet, 363*, 2063–2072.

Mufson, L., & Fairbanks, J. (1996). Interpersonal psychotherapy for depressed adolescents: A one-year naturalistic follow-up study. *Journal of the American Academy of Child & Adolescent Psychiatry, 35*, 1145–1155.

Mufson, L., Gallagher, T., Dorta, K. P., & Young, J. F. (2004). A group adaptation of interpersonal psychotherapy for depressed adolescents. *American Journal of Psychotherapy, 58*, 220–237.

Mufson, L., Moreau, D., Weissman, M. M., & Klerman, G. (1993). *Interpersonal psychotherapy for depressed adolescents*. New York: Guilford Press.

Mufson, L., Moreau, D., Weissman, M. M., Wickramaratne, P., Martin, J., & Samoilov, A. (1994). Modification of interpersonal psychotherapy with depressed adolescents (IPT-A): Phase I and II studies. *Journal of the American Academy of Child & Adolescent Psychiatry, 3*, 695–705.

Mufson, L., Weissman, M. M., Moreau, D., & Garfinkel, R. (1999). Efficacy of interpersonal psychotherapy for depressed adolescents. *Archives of General Psychiatry, 56*, 573–579.

Multimodal Treatment of ADHD Cooperative Group. (1999a). 14-month randomized clinical trial of treatment strategies for attention-deficit/hyperactivity disorder. *Archives of General Psychiatry, 56*, 1073–1086.

Multimodal Treatment of ADHD Cooperative Group. (1999b). Moderators and mediators of treatment response for children with attention-deficit/hyperactivity disorder. *Archives of General Psychiatry, 56*, 1088–1096.

Multimodal Treatment of ADHD Cooperative Group. (2004a). National Institute of Mental Health multimodal treatment study of ADHD follow-up: Changes in effectiveness and growth after the end of treatment. *Pediatrics, 113*, 762–769.

Multimodal Treatment of ADHD Cooperative Group. (2004b). National Institute of Mental Health multimodal treatment study of ADHD follow-up: 24-month outcomes of treatment strategies for attention-deficit/hyperactivity disorder. *Pediatrics, 113*, 754–761.

Multimodal Treatment of ADHD Cooperative Group. (2007). *3-year follow-up of the NIMH MTA study*. Manuscript submitted for publication.

Muñoz, C., & Hilgenberg, C. (2005). Ethnopharmacology. *American Journal of Nursing, 105*, 40–48.

Muñoz, R. F., Hollon, S. D., McGrath, E., Rehm, L. P., & VandenBos, G. R. (1994). On the AHCPR depression in primary care guidelines: Further considerations for practitioners. *American Psychologist, 49*, 42–61.

Myers, K., McCauley, E., Calderon, R., & Treder, R. (1991). The 3-year longitudinal course of suicidality and predictive factors for subsequent suicidality in youths with major depressive disorder. *Journal of the American Academy of Child & Adolescent Psychiatry, 30*, 804–810.

National Center for Health Statistics. (2004). *Health, United States, 2004: With chartbook on trends in the health of Americans*. Washington, DC: U.S. Government Printing Office.

National Institutes of Health. (1998). *National Institutes of Health consensus statement: Diagnosis and treatment of attention deficit hyperactivity disorder*. Bethesda, MD: Author.

National Research Council. (2001). *Educating children with autism*. Washington, DC: National Academy Press.

Nauta, M., Scholing, A., Emmelkamp, P., & Minderaa, R. (2003). Cognitive–behavioral therapy for children with anxiety disorders in a clinical setting: No additional effect of a cognitive parent training. *Journal of the American Academy of Child & Adolescent Psychiatry, 42*, 1270–1278.

Newcorn, J. H., Spencer, T. J., Biederman, J., Milton, D. R., & Michelson, D. (2005). Atomoxetine treatment in children and adolescents with attention-deficit/hyperactivity disorder and comorbid oppositional defiant disorder. *Journal of the American Academy of Child & Adolescent Psychiatry, 44*, 240–248.

Noell, G. H., Witt, J. C., Slider, N. J., Connell, J. E., Gatti, S. L., Williams, K. L., et al. (2005). Treatment implementation following behavioral consultation in schools: A comparison of three follow-up strategies. *School Psychology Review, 34*, 87–106.

Northup, J., Fusilier, I., Swanson, V., Huerte, J., Bruce, T., Freeland, J., et al. (1999). Further analysis of the separate and interactive effects of methylphenidate and common classroom contingencies. *Journal of Applied Behavior Analysis, 32*, 35–50.

O'Leary, K. D., Pelham, W. E., Rosenbaum, A., & Price, G. H. (1976). Behavioral treatment of hyperkinetic children: An experimental evaluation of its usefulness. *Clinical Pediatrics, 15*, 510–515.

O'Leary, S. G. (1980). Skills or pills for hyperactive children. *Journal of Applied Behavioral Analysis, 13*, 191–204.

O'Leary, S. G., & Pelham, W. E. (1978). Behavior therapy and withdrawal of stimulant medication in hyperactive children. *Pediatrics, 61*, 211–217.

Olfson, M., Gameroff, M. J., Marcus, S. C., & Jensen, P. S. (2003). National trends in the treatment of attention deficit hyperactivity disorder. *American Journal of Psychiatry, 160*, 1071–1077.

Olfson, M., Gameroff, M. J., Marcus, S. C., & Waslick, B. D. (2003). Outpatient treatment of child and adolescent depression in the United States. *Archives of General Psychiatry, 60*, 1236–1242.

Olfson, M., Marcus, S. C., & Schaffer, D. (2006). Antidepressant drug therapy and suicide in severly depressed children and adults. *Archives of General Psychiatry, 63*, 865–872.

Olfson, M., Marcus, S. C., Weissman, M. M., & Jensen, P. S. (2002). National trends in the use of psychotropic medications by children. *Journal of the American Academy of Child & Adolescent Psychiatry, 41*, 514–521.

Ondersma, S. J., & Walker, C. E. (1998). Elimination disorders. In T. H. Ollendick & M. Hersen (Eds.), *Handbook of child psychopathology* (3rd ed., pp. 355–380). New York: Plenum Press.

Ost, L. G., Svensson, L., Hellstrom, K., & Lindwall, R. (2001). One-session treatment of specific phobias in youths: A randomized clinical trial. *Journal of Consulting and Clinical Psychology, 69*, 814–824.

Ota, K. R., & DuPaul, G. J. (2002). Task engagement and mathematics performance in children with attention-deficit hyperactivity disorder: Effects of supplemental computer instruction. *School Psychology Quarterly, 17*, 242–257.

Palumbo, D., Sallee, F., Pelham, W., Bukstein, O., McDermott, M., & The CAT Study Group. (2005, October). *Clonidine in attention treatment: Primary outcomes.* Poster presented at the annual meeting of the American Academy of Child & Adolescent Psychiatry, Toronto, Ontario, Canada.

Palumbo, D., Spencer, T., Lynch, J., Co-Chien, H., & Faraone, S. V. (2004). Emergence of tics in children with ADHD: Impact of once-daily OROS methylphenidate therapy. *Journal of Child and Adolescent Psychopharmacology, 14*, 185–194.

Papatheodorou, G., & Kutcher, S. P. (1993). Divalproex sodium treatment in late adolescent and young adult acute mania. *Psychopharmacology Bulletin, 29*, 213–219.

Papatheodorou, G., Kutcher, S. P., Katic, M., & Szalai, J. P. (1995). The efficacy and safety of divalproex sodium in the treatment of acute mania in adolescents and young adults: An open clinical trial. *Journal of Clinical Psychopharmacology, 15*, 110–116.

Pavuluri, M. N., Graczyk, P. A., Henry, D. B., Carbray, J. A., Heidenreich, J., & Miklowitz, D. J. (2004). Child- and family-focused cognitive behavioral therapy for pediatric bipolar disorder: Development and preliminary results. *Journal of the American Academy of Child & Adolescent Psychiatry, 43*, 528–537.

Paykel, E. S., Hart, D., & Priest, R. G. (1998). Changes in public attitudes to depression during the Defeat Depression Campaign. *British Journal of Psychiatry, 173*, 519–522.

Pediatric OCD Treatment Study Team. (2004). Cognitive–behavioral therapy, sertraline, and their combination for children and adolescents with obsessive–compulsive disorder: The Pediatric OCD Treatment Study (POTS) randomized controlled trial. *Journal of the American Medical Association, 292,* 1969–1976.

Pelham, W. E., Burrows-MacLean, L., Gnagy, E. M., Arnold, F., Chacko, A., Coles, E. K., et al. (2007). *A dose ranging study of behavioral and pharmacological treatment in recreational settings for children with ADHD.* Manuscript submitted for publication.

Pelham, W. E., Burrows-MacLean, L., Gnagy, E. M., Fabiano, G. A., Coles, E. K., Tresco, K. E., et al. (2005). Transdermal methylphenidate, behavioral, and combined treatment for children with ADHD. *Experimental and Clinical Psychopharmacology, 13,* 111–126.

Pelham, W. E., Carlson, C., Sams, S. E., Vallano, G., Dixon, M. J., & Hoza, B. (1993). Separate and combined effects of methylphenidate and behavior modification on boys with attention deficit–hyperactivity disorder in a classroom. *Journal of Consulting and Clinical Psychology, 61,* 506–515.

Pelham, W. E., Erhardt, D., Gnagy, E. M., Greiner, A. R., Arnold, L. E., Abikoff, H. B., et al. (2007). *Parent and teacher evaluation of treatment in the* MTA: *Consumer satisfaction and perceived effectiveness.* Manuscript submitted for publication.

Pelham, W. E., & Fabiano, G. A. (in press). Evidence-based psychosocial treatment for attention-deficit/hyperactivity disorder: An update. *Journal of Clinical Child and Adolescent Psychology.*

Pelham, W. E., Fabiano, G. A., Gnagy, E. M., Greiner, A. R., Hoza, B., Manos, M., & Janakovic, F. (2005). Comprehensive psychosocial treatment for ADHD. In E. Hibbs & P. Jensen (Eds.), *Psychosocial treatments for child and adolescent disorders: Empirically based strategies for clinical practice* (2nd ed., pp. 377–410). Washington, DC: American Psychological Association.

Pelham, W. E., Fabiano, G. A., & Massetti, G. M. (2005). Evidence-based assessment of attention-deficit/hyperactivity disorder in children and adolescents. *Journal of Clinical Child and Adolescent Psychology, 34,* 449–476.

Pelham, W. E., Gnagy, E. M., Arnold, F., Burrows-MacLean, L., Chacko, A., Coles, E. K., et al. (2007). *A between-group study of intensity of behavioral treatment and dose of methylphenidate in ADHD.* Manuscript submitted for publication.

Pelham, W. E., Gnagy, E. M., Greiner, A. R., Hoza, B., Hinshaw, S. P., Swanson, J. M., et al. (2000). Behavioral versus behavioral and pharmacological treatment in ADHD children attending a summer treatment program. *Journal of Abnormal Child Psychology, 28,* 507–526.

Pelham, W. E., & Hoza, B. (1996). Intensive treatment: A summer treatment program for children with ADHD. In E. Hibbs & P. Jensen (Eds.), *Psychosocial treatments for child and adolescent disorders: Empirically based strategies for clinical practice* (pp. 311–340). Washington, DC: American Psychological Association.

Pelham, W. E., Molina, B. S., Gnagy, E. M., Meichenbaum, D. L., & Greenhouse, J. B. (2007). *The impact of childhood stimulant medication on later substance use.* Manuscript submitted for publication.

Pelham, W. E., Schnedler, R. W., Bender, M. E., Miller, J., Nilsson, D., Budrow, M., et al. (1988). The combination of behavior therapy and methylphenidate in the treatment of hyperactivity: A therapy outcome study. In L. Bloomingdale (Ed.), *Attention deficit disorders* (Vol. III, pp. 29–48). London: Pergamon Press.

Pelham, W. E., Schnedler, R. W., Bologna, N. C., & Contreras, J. A. (1980). Behavioral and stimulant treatment of hyperactive children: A therapy study with methylphenidate probes in a within-subject design. *Journal of Applied Behavior Analysis, 13,* 221–236.

Pelham, W. E., Vodde-Hamilton, M., Murphy, D. A., Greenstein, J. L., & Vallano, G. (1991). The effects of methylphenidate on ADHD adolescents in recreational, peer group, and classroom settings. *Journal of Clinical Child Psychology, 20,* 293–300.

Pelham, W. E., Walker, J. L., Sturges, J., & Hoza, J. (1989). The comparative effects of methylphenidate on ADD girls and ADD boys. *Journal of the American Academy of Child & Adolescent Psychiatry, 28,* 773–776.

Pelham, W. E., & Waschbusch, D. A. (1999). Behavioral interventions in attention-deficit/hyperactivity disorder. In H. Quay & A. Hogan (Eds.), *Handbook of disruptive behavior disorders* (pp. 255–278). New York: Kluwer Academic/Plenum Publishers.

Pelham, W. E., Wheeler, T., & Chronis, A. M. (1998). Empirically supported psychosocial treatments for ADHD. *Journal of Child Clinical Psychology, 27,* 189–204.

Penn, D. L., Waldheter, E. J., Perkins, D. O., Mueser, K. T., & Lieberman, J. A. (2005). Psychosocial treatment for first-episode psychosis: A research update. *American Journal of Psychiatry, 162,* 2220–2232.

Petersen, A. C., Compas, B. E., Brooks-Gunn, J., Stemmler, M., Ey, S., & Grant, K. E. (1993). Depression during adolescence. *American Psychologist, 48,* 155–168.

Peterson, A. A., Campise, R., & Azrin, N. (1994). Behavioral and pharmacological treatments for tic and habit disorders: A review. *Developmental and Behavioral Pediatrics, 15,* 430–441.

Peterson, A. L. (2007). Psychosocial management of tics and intentional repetitive behaviors associated with Tourette Syndrome. In D. W. Woods, J. C. Piacentini, & J. T. Walkup (Eds.), *Treating Tourette Syndrome and tic disorders: A guide for practitioners* (pp. 154–184). New York: Guilford Press.

Pfiffner, L .J., & McBurnett, K. (1997). Social skills training with parent generalization: Treatment effects for children with attention deficit disorder. *Journal of Consulting and Clinical Psychology, 65,* 749–757.

Phelps, L., Brown, R. T., & Power, T. (2002). *Pediatric psychopharmacology: Combining medical and psychosocial interventions.* Washington, DC: American Psychological Association.

Piacentini, J., (2004, July). *Controlled comparison of CBT and relaxation training for childhood OCD.* Paper presented at the annual convention of the American Psychological Association, Honolulu, HI.

Piacentini, J., Bergman, R. L., Keller, M., & McCracken, J. (2003). Functional impairment in children and adolescents with obsessive compulsive disorder. *Journal of Child and Adolescent Psychopharmacology, 13,* 61–70.

Piacentini, J., & Chang, S. (2001). Behavioral treatments for Tourette syndrome and tic disorders: State of the art. In D. J. Cohen, C. G. Goetz, & J. Jankovic (Eds.), *Advances in Neurology: Vol. 85. Tourette syndrome* (pp. 319–331). Philadelphia: Lippincott Williams & Wilkins.

Piacentini, J., & Chang, S. (2006). Behavioral treatments for tic suppression: Habit reversal therapy. In J. Walkup, J. Mink, & P. Hollenbeck (Eds.), *Advances in neurology: Tourette syndrome* (pp. 227–233). Philadelphia: Lippincott Williams & Wilkins.

Piacentini, J., & Langley, A. (2004). Cognitive–behavioral therapy for children who have obsessive–compulsive disorder. *Journal of Clinical Psychology, 60,* 1181–1194.

Piacentini, J., March, J., & Franklin, M. (2006). Cognitive–behavioral therapy for youngsters with obsessive–compulsive disorder. In P. Kendall (Ed.), *Child and adolescent therapy: Cognitive–behavioral procedures* (3rd ed., pp. 297–321). New York: Guilford Press.

Pike, K. M., & Striegel-Moore, R. H. (1997). Disordered eating and eating disorders. In S. J. Gallant, G. P. Keita, & R. Royak-Schaler (Eds.), *Health care for women: Psychological, social, and behavioral sciences* (pp. 97–114). Washington, DC: American Psychological Association.

Pina, A. A., Silverman, W. K., Fuentes, R. M., Kurtines, W. M., & Weems, C. F. (2003). Exposure-based cognitive–behavioral treatment for phobic and anxiety disorders: Treatment effects and maintenance for Hispanic/Latino relative to European-American youths. *Journal of the American Academy of Child & Adolescent Psychiatry, 42,* 1179–1187.

Pine, D. S. (1994). Child–adult anxiety disorders. *Journal of the American Academy of Child & Adolescent Psychiatry, 33,* 280–281.

Pisterman, S., McGrath, P., Firestone, P., Goodman, J. T., Webster, I., & Mallory, R. (1989). Outcome of parent-medicated treatment with preschoolers with attention deficit disorder with hyperactivity. *Journal of Consulting and Clinical Psychology, 57,* 628–635.

Posey, D. J., & McDougle, C. J. (2001). Pharmacotherapeutic management of autism. *Expert Opinions in Pharmacotherapy, 2,* 587–600.

Preda, A., MacLean, R. W., Mazure, C. M., & Bowers, M. B. (2001). Antidepressant-associated mania and psychosis resulting in psychiatric admissions. *Journal of Clinical Psychiatry, 62,* 30–33.

Priest, R. G., Vize, C., Roberts, A., Roberts, M., & Tylee, A. (1996). Lay people's attitude to treatment of depression: Results of opinion poll for Defeat Depression Campaign just before its launch. *British Medical Journal, 313,* 858–859.

Prince, J. B., Wilens, T. E., Biederman, J., Spencer, T. J., & Wozniak, J. R. (1996). Clonidine for sleep disturbances associated with attention-deficit hyperactivity disorder: A systematic chart review of 62 cases. *Journal of the American Academy of Child & Adolescent Psychiatry, 35*, 599–605.

Puig-Antich, J., Kaufman, J., Ryan, N. D., Williamson, D. E., Dahl, R. E., Lukens, E., et al. (1993). The psychosocial functioning and family environment of depressed adolescents. *Journal of the American Academy of Child & Adolescent Psychiatry, 32*, 244–253.

Rao, U., Weissman, M. M., Martin, J. A., & Hammond, R. W. (1993). Childhood depression and risk of suicide: A preliminary report of a longitudinal study. *Journal of the American Academy of Child & Adolescent Psychiatry, 32*, 21–27.

Rapoport, J., Inoff-Germain, G., Weissman, M. M., Greenwald, S., Narrow, W. E., Jensen, P. S., et al. (2000). Childhood obsessive–compulsive disorder in the NIMH MECA study: Parent versus child identification of cases. *Journal of Anxiety Disorders, 14*, 535–548.

Rapport, M. D., & Denney, C. B. (2000). Attention deficit hyperactivity disorder and methylphenidate: Assessment and prediction of clinical response. In L. L. Greenhill & B. B. Osman (Eds.), *Ritalin: Theory and practice* (2nd ed., pp. 45–70). Larchmont, NY: Mary Ann Liebert.

Remschmidt, H. E., Hennighausen, K., Clement, H. W., Heiser, P., & Schultz, E. (2000). Atypical neuroleptics in child and adolescent psychiatry. *European Child and Adolescent Psychiatry,* 9(Suppl. 1), I9–I19.

Research Units on Pediatric Psychopharmacology Anxiety Study Group. (2001a). An eight-week placebo-controlled trial of fluvoxamine for anxiety disorders in children and adolescents. *New England Journal of Medicine, 344*, 1279–1285.

Research Units on Pediatric Psychopharmacology Anxiety Study Group. (2001b). Fluvoxamine for the treatment of anxiety disorders in children and adolescents. *New England Journal of Medicine, 344*, 1279–1285.

Research Units on Pediatric Psychopharmacology Anxiety Study Group. (2002). Treatment of pediatric anxiety disorders: An open-label extension of the Research Units on Pediatric Psychopharmacology Anxiety Study. *Journal of Child and Adolescent Psychopharmacology, 12*, 175–188.

Research Units on Pediatric Psychopharmacology Anxiety Study Group. (2003). Searching for moderators and mediators of pharmacological treatment effects in children and adolescents with anxiety disorders. *Journal of the American Academy of Child & Adolescent Psychiatry, 42*, 13–21.

Research Units on Pediatric Psychopharmacology Autism Network. (2002). Risperidone in children with autism and serious behavioral problems. *New England Journal of Medicine, 347*, 314–321.

Research Units on Pediatric Psychopharmacology Autism Network. (2005a). A randomized, double-blind, placebo-controlled, crossover trial of methylphenidate in children with hyperactivity associated with pervasive developmental disorders. *Archives of General Psychiatry, 62*, 1266–1274.

Research Units on Pediatric Psychopharmacology Autism Network. (2005b). Risperidone treatment of autistic disorder: Longer term benefits and blinded discontinuation after six months. *American Journal of Psychiatry, 162*, 1361–1369.

Reyno, S. M., & McGrath, P. J. (2006). Predictors of parent training efficacy for child externalizing behavior problems: A meta-analytic review. *Journal of Child Psychology and Psychiatry and Allied Disciplines, 47*, 99–111.

Reynolds, W. M., & Coats, K. I. (1986). A comparison of cognitive–behavioral therapy and relaxation training for the treatment of depression in adolescents. *Journal of Consulting and Clinical Psychology, 44*, 653–660.

Rigoni, G. (2004, February 2). *Drug utilization for selected antidepressants among children and adolescents in the U.S.* Retrieved April 22, 2005, from http://www.fda.gov/ohrms/dockets/ac/04/slides040061.htm

Roberts, R. E., Atkinson, C. C., & Rosenblatt, A. (1998). Prevalence of psychopathology among children and adolescents. *American Journal of Psychiatry, 155*, 715–725.

Robin, A. L., Siegel, P. T., Moye, A. W., Gilroy, M., Dennis, A. B., & Sikand, A. (1999). A controlled comparison of family versus individual therapy for adolescents with anorexia nervosa. *Journal of the American Academy of Child & Adolescent Psychiatry, 38*, 1482–1489.

Robison, L. M., Sclar, D. A., Skaer, T. L., & Galin, R. S. (2004). Treatment modalities among U.S. children diagnosed with attention-deficit hyperactivity disorder: 1995–1999. *International Clinical Psychopharmacology, 19*, 17–22.

Rogers, S. J., & Lewis, H. (1989). An effective day treatment model for young children with pervasive developmental disorders. *Journal of the American Academy of Child & Adolescent Psychiatry, 28*, 207–214.

Rohde, P., Clarke, G. N., Lewinsohn, P. M., Seeley J. R., & Kaufman N. K. (2001). Impact of comorbidity on a cognitive–behavioral group treatment for adolescent depression. *Journal of the American Academy of Child & Adolescent Psychiatry, 40*, 795–802.

Rohde, P., Clarke, G. N., Mace, D. E., Jorgensen, J. S., & Seeley, J. R. (2004). An efficacy/effectiveness study of cognitive–behavioral treatment for adolescents with comorbid major depression and conduct disorder. *Journal of the American Academy of Child & Adolescent Psychiatry, 43*, 660–668.

Rohde, P., Lewinsohn, P. M., & Clarke, G. N. (2005). The adolescent coping with depression course: A cognitive–behavioral approach to the treatment of adolescent depression. In. E. D. Hibbs & P. S. Jensen (Eds.), *Psychosocial treatments for child and adolescent disorders: Empirically based strategies for clinical practice* (pp. 219–237). Washington, DC: American Psychological Association.

Root, R., & Resnick, R. (2003). An update on the diagnosis and treatment of attention-deficit/hyperactivity disorder in children. *Professional Psychology: Research and Practice, 34*, 34–41.

Rosenbaum, J. F., Fava, M., Hoog, S. L., Ashcroft, R. C., & Krebs, W. B. (1998). Selective serotonin reuptake inhibitor discontinuation syndrome: A randomized clinical trial. *Biological Psychiatry, 44*, 77–87.

Rosselló, J., & Bernal, G. (1999). The efficacy of cognitive–behavioral and interpersonal treatments for depression in Puerto Rican adolescents. *Journal of Consulting and Clinical Psychology, 67,* 734–745.

Rotheram-Borus, M. J., Piacentini, J., Cantwell, C., Belin, T. R., & Song, J. (2000). The 18-month impact of an emergency room intervention for adolescent female suicide attempters. *Journal of Consulting and Clinical Psychology, 88,* 1081–1093.

Rotheram-Borus, M. J., Piacentini, J., VanRossem, R., Graae, F., Cantwell, C., Castro-Blanco, D., et al. (1996). Enhancing treatment adherence with a specialized emergency room program for adolescent suicide attempters. *Journal of the American Academy of Child & Adolescent Psychiatry, 35,* 655–663.

Russell, G. F., Szmukler, G. I., Dare, C., & Eisler, I. (1987). An evaluation of family therapy in anorexia nervosa and bulimia nervosa. *Archives of General Psychiatry, 44,* 1047–1056.

Rynn, M. A., Siqueland, L., & Rickels, K. (2001). Placebo-controlled trial of sertraline in the treatment of children with generalized anxiety disorder. *American Journal of Psychiatry, 158,* 2008–2014.

Sackett, D., Richardson, W., Rosemberg, W., & Haynes, B. (2000). *Evidence-based medicine* (2nd ed.). London: Churchill Livingstone.

Safer, D. J., & Zito, J. M. (2000). Pharmacoepidemiology of methylphenidate and other stimulants for the treatment of attention deficit hyperactivity disorder. In L. L. Greenhill & B. B. Osman (Eds.), *Ritalin: Theory and practice* (2nd ed., pp. 7–26). Larchmont, NY: Mary Ann Liebert.

Safer, D. J., Zito, J. M., & DosReis, S. (2003). Concomitant psychotropic medication for youths. *American Journal of Psychiatry, 160,* 438–449.

Sallee, F. R., Kurlan, R., Goetz, C., Singer, H., Scahill, L., Law, G., et al. (2000). Ziprasidone treatment of children and adolescents with Tourette's syndrome: A pilot study. *Journal of the American Academy of Child & Adolescent Psychiatry, 39,* 292–299.

Sallee, F. R., Nesbitt, L., Jackson, C., Sine, L., & Sethuraman, G. (1997). Relative efficacy of haloperidol and pimozide in children with Tourette syndrome with and without attention deficit hyperactivity disorder. *Journal of American Psychiatry, 154,* 1057–1062.

Sandler, A. D., Sutton, K. A., DeWeese, J., Girardi, M. A., Sheppard, V., & Bodfish, J. W. (1999). Lack of benefit of a single dose of synthetic human secretin in the treatment of autism and pervasive developmental disorder. *New England Journal of Medicine, 341,* 1801–1806.

Sandor, P. (2003). Pharmacological management of tics in patients with TS. *Journal of Psychosomatic Research, 55,* 41–48.

Scahill, L., Chappell, P., Kim, Y. S., Schultz, R., Katsovich, L., Shepherd, E., et al. (2001). A placebo-controlled study of guanfacine in the treatment of children with tic disorders and attention deficit hyperactivity disorder. *American Journal of Psychiatry, 158,* 1067–1074.

Scahill, L., Chappell, P., King, R., & Leckman, J. (2000). Pharmacologic treatment of tic disorders. *Psychopharmacology*, 9, 99–117.

Scahill, L., Sukhodolsky, D., Williams, S., & Leckman, J. (2005). Public health significance of tic disorders in children and adolescents. *Advances in Neurology*, 96, 240–248.

Schopler, E., & Mesibov, G. (Eds.). (1995). *Learning and cognition in autism*. New York: Plenum.

Shaffer, D., Fisher, P., Dulcan, M. K., & Davies, M. (1996). The NIMH Diagnostic Interview Schedule for Children Version 2.3 (DISC—2.3): Description, acceptability, prevalence rates, and performance in the MECA study. *Journal of the American Academy of Child & Adolescent Psychiatry*, 35, 865–877.

Shaffer, D., Garland, A., Gould, M., Fisher, P., & Trautman, P. (1988). Preventing teenage suicide: A critical review. *Journal of the American Academy of Child & Adolescent Psychiatry*, *27*, 675–687.

Shapiro, E., Shapiro, A., Fulop, G., Hubbard, M., Mandeli, J., Nordlie, J., & Phillips, R. (1989). Controlled study of haloperidol, pimozide and placebo for the treatment of Gilles de la Tourette's syndrome. *Archives of General Psychiatry*, *46*, 722–730.

Sharpe, C. R., Collet, J. P., Belzile, E., Hanley, J. A., & Boivin, J. F. (2002). The effects of tricyclic antidepressants on breast cancer risk. *British Journal of Cancer*, 86, 92–97.

Shea, S., Turgay, A., Carroll, A., Schultz, M., Orlik, H., Smith, I., et al. (2004). Risperidone in the treatment of disruptive behavioral symptoms in children with autistic and other pervasive developmental disorders. *Pediatrics*, *114*, e634–e641.

Sikich, L., Hamer, R. M., Bashford, R. A., Sheitman, B. B., & Lieberman, J. A. (2004). A pilot study of risperidone, olanzapine, and haloperidol in psychotic youth: A double-blind, randomized, 8-week trial. *Neuropsychopharmacology*, *29*, 133–145.

Silverman, W. K., & Berman, S. L. (2001). Psychosocial interventions for anxiety disorders in children: Status and future directions. In W. K. Silverman & P. D. A. Treffers (Eds.), *Anxiety disorders in children and adolescents: Research, assessment and intervention* (pp. 313–334). New York: Cambridge University Press

Silverman, W. K., Kurtines, W. M., Ginsburg, G. S., Weems, C. F., Lumpkin, P. W., & Carmichael, D. H. (1999). Treating anxiety disorders in children with group cognitive–behavioral therapy: A randomized clinical trial. *Journal of Consulting and Clinical Psychology*, *67*, 995–1003.

Silverman, W. K., Kurtines, W. M., Ginsburg, G. S., Weems, C. F., Rabian, B., & Serafini, L. T. (1999). Contingency management, self-control, and education support in the treatment of childhood phobic disorders: A randomized clinical trial. *Journal of Consulting and Clinical Psychology*, *67*, 675–687.

Simeon, J., Dinicola, V., Ferguson, B., & Copping, W. (1990). Adolescent depression: A placebo-controlled fluoxetine treatment study and follow-up. *Progress in Neuro-psychopharmacology and Biological Psychiatry*, *14*, 791–795.

Simmonds, S., Coid, J., Joseph, P., Marriott, S., & Tyler, P. (2001). Community mental health team management in severe mental illness: A systematic review. *British Journal of Psychiatry, 17*, 497–502.

Singer, H., Brown, J., Quaskey, S., Rosenberg, L., Mellits, E., & Denckla, M. (1995). The treatment of attention-deficit hyperactivity disorder in Tourette's syndrome: A double-blind placebo-controlled study with clonidine and desipramine. *Pediatrics, 95*, 74–81.

Smith, B. H., Pelham, W. E., Evans, S., Gnagy, E., Molina, B., Bukstein, O., et al. (1998). Dosage effects of methylphenidate on the social behavior of adolescents diagnosed with attention-deficit hyperactivity disorder. *Experimental and Clinical Psychopharmacology*, 6, 187–204.

Smith, B. H., Waschbusch, D. A., Willoughby, M. T., & Evans, S. (2000). The efficacy, safety and practicality of treatments for adolescents with attention-deficit/hyperactivity disorder (ADHD). *Clinical Child and Family Psychology Review, 3*, 243–267.

Smith, T., Groen, A. D., & Wynn, J. W. (2000). Randomized trial of intensive early intervention for children with pervasive developmental disorder. *American Journal on Mental Retardation, 105*, 269–285.

Snyder, R., Turgay, A., Aman, M., Binder, C., Fisman, S., Carroll, A., & Risperidone Conduct Study Group. (2002). Effects of risperidone on conduct and disruptive behavior disorders in children with subaverage IQs. *Journal of the American Academy of Child & Adolescent Psychiatry, 41*, 1026–1036.

Sommers-Flanagan, J., & Sommers-Flanagan, R. (1996). Efficacy of antidepressant medication with depressed youth: What psychologists should know. *Professional Psychology: Research and Practice, 27*, 145–153.

Sonuga-Barke, E. J. S., Daley, D., Thompson, M., Laver-Bradbury, C., & Weeks, A. (2001). Parent-based therapies for preschool attention-deficit/hyperactivity disorder: A randomized, controlled trial with a community sample. *Journal of the American Academy of Child & Adolescent Psychiatry, 40*, 402–408.

Southam-Gerow, M., Weisz, J., & Kendall, P. C. (2003). Youth with anxiety disorders in research and service clinics: Examining client differences and similarities. *Journal of Clinical Child and Adolescent Psychology, 32*, 375–385.

Spence, S. H., Donovan, C., & Brechman-Toussaint, M. (2000). The treatment of childhood social phobia: The effectiveness of a social skills training-based, cognitive–behavioural intervention, with and without parental involvement. *Journal of Child Psychology and Psychiatry, 41*, 713–726.

Spencer, T. J., Biederman, J., & Wilens, T. (1998). Pharmacotherapy of ADHD with antidepressants. In R. A. Barkley (Ed.), *Attention-deficit hyperactivity disorder: A handbook for diagnosis and treatment* (2nd ed., pp. 552–563). New York: Guilford Press.

Spencer, T. J., Biederman, J., Wilens, T., Harding, M., O'Donnell, D., & Griffin, S. (1996). Pharmacotherapy of ADHD across the life cycle. *Journal of the American Academy of Child & Adolescent Psychiatry, 35*, 409–432.

Spencer, T. J., Biederman, J., Wilens, T., Steingard, R., & Geist, D. (1993). Nortriptyline in the treatment of children with attention-deficit hyperactivity disorder and tic disorder or Tourette's syndrome. *Journal of the American Academy of Child & Adolescent Psychiatry, 32,* 205–210.

Stark, K. D., Reynolds, W. M., & Kaslow, N. J. (1987). A comparison of the relative efficacy of self-control therapy and a behavioral problem-solving therapy for depression in children. *Journal of Abnormal Child Psychology, 15,* 91–113.

Stein, B. D., Jaycox, L. H., Kataoka, S. H., Wong, M., Tu, W., Elliott, M. N., & Fink, A. (2003). A mental health intervention for schoolchildren exposed to violence: A randomized controlled trial. *Journal of the American Medical Association, 290,* 603–611.

Steiner, H., Petersen, M. L., Saxena, K., Ford, S., & Matthews, Z. (2003). Divalproex sodium for the treatment of conduct disorder: A randomized controlled clinical trial. *Journal of Clinical Psychiatry, 64,* 1183–1191.

Sterling-Turner, H. E., Watson, T. S., & Moore, J. W. (2002). The effects of direct training and treatment integrity on treatment outcomes in school consultation. *School Psychology Quarterly, 17,* 47–77.

Stevens, J., Harman, J. S., & Kelleher, K. J. (2005). Race/ethnicity and insurance status as factors associated with ADHD treatment patterns. *Journal of Child and Adolescent Psychopharmacology, 15,* 88–96.

Stewart, S., Geller, D., Jenike, M., Pauls, D., Shaw, D., Mullin, B., & Faraone, S. (2004). Long-term outcome of pediatric obsessive–compulsive disorder: A meta-analysis and qualitative review of the literature. *Acta Psychiatrica Scandinavica, 110,* 4–13.

Strickland, T., Lin, K. M., Fu, P., Anderson, D., & Zheng, Y. P. (1995). Comparison of lithium ratio between African American and Caucasian bipolar patients. *Biological Psychiatry, 37,* 325–330.

Strober, M., Freeman, R., DeAntonio, M., Lampert, C., & Diamond, J. (1997). Does adjunctive fluoxetine influence the post-hospital course of restrictor-type anorexia nervosa? A 24-month prospective, longitudinal followup and comparison with historical controls. *Psychopharmacology Bulletin, 33,* 425–431.

Sturmey, P. (2005). Secretin is an ineffective treatment for pervasive developmental disabilities: A review of 15 double-blind randomized controlled trials. *Research in Developmental Disabilities, 26,* 87–97.

Swanson, J. M., Elliott, G. R., Greenhill, L. L., Stehli, A., Arnold, L. E., Epstein, J., et al. (2007). *Effects of stimulant medication on growth rates across 3 years in the MTA follow-up.* Manuscript submitted for publication.

Swanson, J. M., Kraemer, H. C., Hinshaw, S. P., Arnold, L. E., Conners, C. K., Abikoff, H. B., et al. (2001). Clinical relevance of the primary findings of the MTA: Success rates based on severity of ADHD and ODD symptoms at the end of treatment. *Journal of American Academy of Child & Adolescent Psychiatry, 40,* 168–179.

Swanson, J. M., McBurnett, K., Christian, D. L., & Wigal, T. (1995). Stimulant medications and the treatment of children with ADHD. In T. H. Ollendick & R. J. Prinz (Eds.), *Advances in clinical child psychology* (Vol. 17, pp. 265–322). New York: Plenum Press.

Thomsen, P. H. (1996). Schizophrenia with childhood and adolescent onset: A nationwide register-based study. *Acta Psychiatrica Scandinavica, 94*, 187–193.

Tolan, P. H., & Gorman-Smith, D. (1997). Families and the development of urban children. In H. J. Walberg, O. Reyes, & R. P. Weissberg (Eds.), *Children and youth: Interdisciplinary perspectives* (pp. 67–91). Thousand Oaks, CA: Sage.

Tourette's Syndrome Study Group. (2002). Treatment of ADHD in children with tics: A randomized controlled trial. *Neurology, 58*, 527–535.

Treasure, J., & Schmidt, U. (2003). Treatment overview. In J. Treasure, U. Schmidt, & E. van Furth (Eds.), *Handbook of eating disorders* (2nd ed., pp. 207–217). Chichester, England: Wiley.

Treatment for Adolescent Depression Study (TADS) Team. (2004). Fluoxetine, cognitive–behavioral therapy, and their combination for adolescents with depression. *Journal of the American Medical Association, 292*, 807–820.

Troost, P. W., Lahuis, B. E., Steenhuis, M.-P., Ketelaars, C. E., Builtelaar, J. K., Vann England, H., et al. (2005). Long-term effects of risperidone in children with autism spectrum disorders: A placebo discontinuation study. *Journal of the American Academy of Child & Adolescent Psychiatry, 44*, 1137–1144.

Tumuluru, R. V., Weller, E. B., Fristad, M. A., & Weller, R. A. (2003). Mania in six preschool children. *Journal of Child and Adolescent Psychopharmacology, 13*, 489–494.

U.S. Department of Health and Human Services. (1999). *Mental health: A report of the Surgeon General.* Rockville, MD: U.S. Department of Health and Human Services, Substance Abuse and Mental Health Services Administration, Center for Mental Health Services, National Institutes of Health, and National Institute of Mental Health.

U.S. Department of Health and Human Services. (2004). *NTP-CERHR expert panel report on the reproductive and developmental toxicity of fluoxetine* (Center for the Evaluation of Risks to Human Reproduction, National Toxicology Program, NTP-CERHR-Fluoxetine-04). Washington, DC: Author.

U.S. Food and Drug Administration. (2005). *FDA issues public health advisory on Strattera (atomoxetine) for attention deficit disorder.* Washington, DC: Author. Available at http://www.fda.gov/bbs/topics/news/2005/new01237.html

U.S. Food and Drug Administration, Center for Drug Evaluation and Research. (2007). *Antidepressant use in children, adolescents, and adults.* Retrieved May 8, 2007, from http://www.fda.gov/cder/drug/antidepressants/labelTemplate.pdf

U.S. Public Health Service. (1999). *The Surgeon General's call to action to prevent suicide.* Washington DC: Department of Health and Human Services.

U.S. Public Health Service. (2000). *Report of the Surgeon General's Conference on Children's Mental Health: A national action agenda.* Washington, DC: Department of Health and Human Services.

Van Hoeken, D., Seidell, J., & Hoek, H. (2003). Epidemiology. In J. Treasure, U. Schmidt, & E. van Furth (Eds.), *Handbook of eating disorders* (2nd ed., pp. 11–34). Chichester, England: Wiley.

Varley, C., & McClellan, J. (1997). Two additional sudden deaths with tricyclic antidepressants. *Journal of the American Academy of Child & Adolescent Psychiatry, 34,* 390–395.

Verdellen, C., Keijsers, G., Cath, D., & Hoogduin, C. A. (2004). Exposure with response prevention versus habit reversal in Tourette's syndrome: A controlled study. *Behaviour Research and Therapy, 42,* 501–511.

Vitiello, B. (2003). Ethical considerations in psychopharmacological research involving children and adolescents. *Psychopharmacology, 171,* 86–91.

Vitiello, B. (2006). An update on publicly funded multisite trials in pediatric psychopharmacology. *Child and Adolescent Psychiatric Clinics of North America, 15,* 1–12.

Vitiello, B., Heiligenstein, J. J., Riddle, M. A., Greenhill, L. L., & Fegert, J. M. (2004). The interface between publicly funded and industry-funded research in pediatric psychopharmacology: Opportunities for integration and collaboration. *Biological Psychiatry, 56,* 3–9.

Vitiello, B., Riddle, M. A., Greenhill, L. L., March, J. S., Levine, J., Schachar, R. J., et al. (2003). How can we improve the assessment of safety in child and adolescent psychopharmacology? *Journal of the American Academy of Child & Adolescent Psychiatry, 42,* 634–641.

Volkmar, F., & Dykens, E. (2002). Mental retardation. In M. Rutter & E. Taylor (Eds.), *Child and adolescent psychiatry: Modern approaches* (4th ed., pp. 697–710). Malden, MA: Blackwell.

Volkow, N., & Insel, T. (2003). What are the long-term effects of methylphenidate treatment. *Biological Psychiatry, 54,* 1307–1309.

Vostanis, P., Feehan, C., Grattan, E., & Bickerton, W. L. (1996). A randomized controlled outpatient trial of cognitive–behavioural treatment for children and adolescents with depression: 9-month follow-up. *Journal of Affective Disorders, 40,* 105–116.

Wagner, K. D., Ambrosini, P., Rynn, M., Wohlberg, C., Yang, R., Greenbaum, M., et al. (2003). Efficacy of sertraline in the treatment of children and adolescents with major depressive disorder. *Journal of the American Medical Association, 290,* 1033–1041.

Wagner, K. D., Berard, R., Stein, M. B., Wetherhold, E., Carpenter, D. J., Perera, P., et al. (2004). A multicenter, randomized, double-blind, placebo-controlled trial of paroxetine in children and adolescents with social anxiety disorder. *Archives of General Psychiatry, 61,* 1153–1162.

Wagner, K. D., Robb, A. S., Findling, R. L., Jin, J., Gutierrez, M. M., & Heydon, W. E. (2004). A randomized, placebo-controlled trial of citalopram for the treatment of major depression in children and adolescents. *American Journal of Psychiatry, 161,* 1079–1083.

Wagner, K. D., Weller, E. B., Carlson, G. A., Sachs, G., Biederman, J., Frazier, J. A., et al. (2002). An open-label trial of divalproex in children and adolescents with bipolar disorder. *Journal of the American Academy of Child & Adolescent Psychiatry, 41,* 1224–1230.

Waid, A., Chandra, R., Gabel, S., & Chapin, D. (1987). Elevation of biofeedback in childhood encopresis. *Journal of Pediatric Gastroenterology and Nutrition*, 6, 554–558.

Walker, H. M., Colvin, G., & Ramsey, E. (1995). *Antisocial behavior in school: Strategies and best practices.* Pacific Grove, CA: Brooks/Cole.

Walker, H. M., Ramsey, E., & Gresham, F. M. (2003–2004, Winter). Heading off disruptive behavior: How early intervention can reduce defiant behavior—and win back teaching time. *American Educator.* Retrieved March 28, 2007, from http://www.aft.org/pubs-reports/american_educator/winter03-04/early_intervention.html

Waters, T., & Barrett, P. (2000). The role of the family in childhood obsessive–compulsive disorder. *Clinical Child and Family Psychology Review, 3*, 173–184.

Webster-Stratton, C. (1994). Advancing videotape parent training: A comparison study. *Journal of Consulting and Clinical Psychology, 62*, 585–593.

Webster-Stratton, C. (1996). Early onset conduct problems: Does gender make a difference? *Journal of Consulting and Clinical Psychology, 64*, 540–551.

Weersing, V. R., & Weisz, J. R. (2002). Community clinic treatment of depressed youth: Benchmarking usual care against CBT clinical trials. *Journal of Consulting and Clinical Psychology, 70*, 299–310.

Weintrob, N., Cohen, D., Klipper-Aurbach, Y., Zadik, Z., & Dickerman, Z. (2002). Decreased growth during therapy with selective serotonin reuptake inhibitors. *Archives of Pediatric and Adolescent Medicine, 156*, 696–791.

Weiss, B., Caron, A., Ball, S., Tapp, J., Johnson, M., & Weisz, J. R. (2005). Iatrogenic effects of group treatment for antisocial youths. *Journal of Consulting and Clinical Psychology, 73*, 1036–1044.

Weiss, B., Catron, T., Harris, V., & Phung, T. M. (1999). The effectiveness of traditional child psychotherapy. *Journal of Consulting and Clinical Psychology, 67*, 82–94.

Weisz, J. R., Donenberg, G. R., Han, S. S., & Weiss, B. (1995). Bridging the gap between lab and clinic in child and adolescent psychotherapy. *Journal of Consulting and Clinical Psychology, 63*, 688–701.

Weisz, J. R., & Jensen, A. L. (2001). Efficacy and effectiveness of psychotherapy with children and adolescents. *European Child and Adolescent Psychiatry, 10*, I12–I18.

Weisz, J. R., Jensen Doss, A., & Hawley, K. M. (2005). Youth psychotherapy outcome research: A review and critique of the evidence base. *Annual Review of Psychology, 56*, 337–363.

Weisz, J. R., McCarty, C. A., & Valeri, S. M. (2006). Effects of psychotherapy for depression in children and adolescents: A meta-analysis. *Psychological Bulletin, 132*, 132–149.

Weisz, J. R., Thurber, C. A., Sweeney, L., Proffitt, V. D., & LeGagnoux, G. L. (1997). Brief treatment of mild-to-moderate child depression using primary and secondary control enhancement training. *Journal of Consulting and Clinical Psychology, 65*, 703–707.

Wells, K. C. (1999). Treatment research at the crossroads: The scientific interface of clinical trials and effectiveness research. *American Journal of Psychiatry, 156,* 5–10.

Wells, K. C., Chi, T. C., Hinshaw, S. P., Epstein, J. N., Pfiffner, L., Nebel-Schwalm, M., et al. (2006). Treatment related changes in objectively measured parenting behaviors in the multimodal treatment study of children with ADHD. *Journal of Consulting and Clinical Psychology, 74,* 649–657.

Wells, K. C., Epstein, J., Hinshaw, S., Conners, C. K., Abikoff, H. B., Abramowitz, A., et al. (2000). Parenting and family stress treatment outcomes in attention deficit hyperactivity disorder (ADHD): An empirical analysis in the MTA study. *Journal of Abnormal Child Psychology, 28,* 543–554.

Wells, K. C., Pelham, W. E., Kotkin, R. A., Hoza, B., Abikoff, H. B., Abramowitz, A., et al. (2000). Psychosocial treatment strategies in the MTA study: Rationale, methods, and critical issues in design and implementation. *Journal of Abnormal Child Psychology, 28,* 483–506.

Werry, J. S., & Aman, M. G. (1999). *Practitioner's guide to psychoactive drugs for children and adolescents* (2nd ed.). New York: Plenum Press.

Werry, J. S., McClellan, J. M., & Chard, L. (1991). Childhood and adolescent schizophrenic, bipolar, and schizoaffective disorders: A clinical and outcome study. *Journal of the American Academy of Child & Adolescent Psychiatry, 30,* 457–465.

West, S. A., Keck, P. E., Jr., McElroy, S. L., Strakowski, S. M., Minnery, K. L., McConville, B. J., & Sorter, M. T. (1994). Open trial of valproate in the treatment of adolescent mania. *Journal of Child and Adolescent Psychopharmacology, 4,* 263–267.

West, S. A., McElroy, S. L., Strakowski, S. M., Keck, P. E., Jr., & McConville, B. J. (1995). Attention deficit hyperactivity disorder in adolescent mania. *American Journal of Psychiatry, 152,* 271–273.

Whittal, M. L., Agras, W. S., & Gould, R. A. (1999). Bulimia nervosa: A meta analysis of psychosocial and pharmacological treatments. *Behavior Therapy, 30,* 117–135.

Whittington, C. J., Kendall, T., Fonagy, P., Cottrell, D., Cotgrove, A., & Boddington, E. (2004). Selective serotonin reuptake inhibitors in childhood depression: Systematic review of published versus unpublished data. *The Lancet, 363,* 1341–1345.

Whittington, C. J., Kendall, T., & Pilling, S. (2005). Are the SSRIs and atypical antidepressants safe and effective for children and adolescents? *Current Opinion in Psychiatry, 18,* 21–25.

Wickstrom, K., Jones, K., LaFleur, L., & Witt, J. (1998). An analysis of treatment integrity in school-based behavioral consultation. *School Psychology Quarterly, 13,* 141–154.

Wigal, S. B., McGough, J. J., McCracken, J. T., Biederman, J., Spencer, T. J., Posner, K. L., et al. (2005). A laboratory school comparison of mixed amphetamine salts extended release (Adderall XR) and atomoxetine (Strattera) in school-aged children with attention deficit/hyperactivity disorder. *Journal of Attention Disorder, 9,* 275–289.

Wilens, T. E., Biederman, J., Forkner, P., Ditterline, J., Morris, M., Moore, H., et al. (2003). Patterns of comorbidity and dysfunction in clinically referred preschool and school-age children with bipolar disorder. *Journal of Child and Adolescent Psychopharmacology, 13*, 495–505.

Witwer, A., & Lecavalier, L. (2005). Treatment rates and patterns in young people with autism spectrum disorders. *Journal of Child and Adolescent Psychopharmacology, 15*, 671–681.

Woo, S. H., & Park, K. H. (2004). Enuresis alarm treatment as a second line to pharmacotherapy in children with monosymptomatic nocturnal enuresis. *Journal of Urology*, 6, 2615–2617.

Wood, A., Harrington, R., & Moore, A. (1996). Controlled trial of a brief cognitive–behavioral intervention in adolescent parents with depressive disorders. *Journal of Child Psychology & Psychiatry, 37*, 737–746.

Wood, A., Trainor, G., Rothwell, J., Moore, A., & Harrington, R. (2001). Randomized trial of group therapy for repeated deliberate self-harm in adolescents. *Journal of the American Academy of Child & Adolescent Psychiatry, 40*, 1246–1253.

Wood, J. J., Piacentini, J., Southam-Gerow, M., Chu, B., & Sigman, M. (2006). Family cognitive behavioral therapy for child anxiety disorders. *Journal of the American Academy of Child & Adolescent Psychiatry, 45*, 314–321.

Yang, Y. Y. (1985). Prophylactic efficacy of lithium and its effective plasma levels in Chinese bipolar patients. *Acta Psychiatrica Scandanavica, 71*, 171–175.

Yeargin-Allsopp, M., Rice, C., Karapurkar, T., Doernberg, N., Boyle, C., & Murphy, C. (2003). Prevalence of autism in a U.S. metropolitan area. *Journal of the American Medical Association, 289*, 49–55.

Youngstrom, E. A., Findling, R. L., Calabrese, J. R., Gracious, B. L., Dementer, C., Bedoya, D. D., & Price, M. (2004). Comparing the diagnostic accuracy of six potential screening instruments for bipolar disorder in youths aged 5 to 17. *Journal of the American Academy of Child & Adolescent Psychiatry, 43*, 847–858.

Zentall, S. S. (1989). Attentional cuing in spelling tasks for hyperactive and comparison regular classroom children. *The Journal of Special Education, 23*, 83–93.

Zinner, S. (2004). Tourette syndrome—Much more than tics. *Contemporary Pediatrics, 21*, 38–49.

Zito, J. M., Sater, D. J., dosRoeis, S., Gardner, J. F., Soeken, K., Boels, M., & Lynch, F. (2002). Rising prevalence of antidepressants among U.S. youths. *Pediatrics, 109*, 721–727.

Zonfrillo, M. R., Penn, J. V., & Henrietta, L. L. (2005, August). Pediatric psychotropic polypharmacy. *Psychiatry, 2*, 14–19.

AUTHOR INDEX

SUBJECT INDEX

ABOUT THE AUTHORS

Ronald T. Brown, PhD, ABPP, is professor of public health, psychology, and pediatrics and is dean of the College of Health Professions at Temple University. Dr. Brown is a diplomate in clinical health psychology of the American Board of Professional Psychology and is a fellow of the American Psychological Association (APA), the American Psychological Society, the Society of Behavioral Medicine, and the National Academy of Neuropsychology. Dr. Brown has been the recipient of numerous grant awards from the National Institutes of Health, the Centers for Disease Control and Prevention, the Department of Defense, and the Office of Special Education and Rehabilitation Services. Dr. Brown currently is the editor of the *Journal of Pediatric Psychology* and serves on the study section of the Behavioral Medicine and Intervention Outcomes of the Center for Scientific Review of the National Institutes of Health. He has published over 200 articles, chapters, and books related to childhood psychopathology and health psychology. He also has served on the editorial boards of 11 journals related to child and adolescent psychopathology. Dr. Brown serves as a liaison to the American Academy of Pediatrics' subcommittee on the assessment and practice guidelines for attention-deficit/hyperactivity disorder, is chair of the Board of Scientific Affairs of the APA, and serves on the Council of Representatives of the APA.

David O. Antonuccio, PhD, ABPP, is a professor in the Department of Psychiatry and Behavioral Sciences at the University of Nevada School of Medicine. He served on the Nevada State Board of Psychological Examiners from 1990 to 1998. A fellow of the American Psychological Association and an ABPP diplomate in clinical psychology, Dr. Antonuccio is internationally known for his work on depression and smoking cessation. His articles on the comparative effects of psychotherapy and pharmacotherapy have received extensive coverage by the national media and are models of careful scholarship. He was named Outstanding Psychologist by the Nevada State Psychological Association (NSPA) in 1993, received an award of achievement in 1999 from NSPA for his work on depression, was awarded the 2000 McReynolds Foundation Psychological Services Award for "outstanding contributions to clinical science," and received the Bud Ogel Award for Distinguished Achievement in Research in 2006 from the Association for Psychologists in Academic Health Settings.

George J. DuPaul, PhD, is professor of school psychology and associate chairperson of the Department of Education and Human Services at Lehigh University. He has extensive experience providing clinical services to children with attention-deficit/hyperactivity disorder (ADHD) and their families as well as consulting with a variety of school districts regarding the management of students with ADHD. He has been an author or coauthor on over 140 journal articles and book chapters related to ADHD and has published 4 books and 2 videos on the assessment and treatment of ADHD. He is currently investigating the effects of early intervention and school-based interventions for students with ADHD as well as the assessment and treatment of college students with ADHD.

Mary A. Fristad, PhD, ABPP, is professor of psychiatry and psychology at the Ohio State University (OSU), where she has been on the faculty since 1986. She is director of Research and Psychological Services in the OSU Division of Child and Adolescent Psychiatry. Dr. Fristad has published over 125 articles and book chapters addressing the assessment and treatment of childhood-onset depression, suicidality, and bipolar disorder. She has edited the *Handbook of Serious Emotional Disturbance in Children and Adolescents* and cowritten *Raising a Moody Child: How to Cope With Depression and Bipolar Disorder*. Dr. Fristad has served on multiple National Institute of Mental Health review committees, the executive board for the American Psychological Association's (APA's) Society of Clinical Child and Adolescent Psychology (Division 53), several APA task forces, and the board of directors for five Web-based education and support groups for children and families with mood disorders. She has been the principal or coprincipal investigator on over two dozen federal, state, and local grants.

Cheryl A. King, PhD, ABPP, is chief psychologist in the Department of Psychiatry at the University of Michigan Medical School, where she also serves as director of the Youth Depression and Suicide Prevention Program. As associate professor in the Department of Psychiatry and Psychology at the University of Michigan, Dr. King has an extensive history of National Institute of Mental Health and private foundation funding for her research with suicidal and depressed adolescents. The author of numerous scientific publications, Dr. King serves on several editorial boards and is a frequent reviewer of grant applications in her area of specialization. Dr. King is past president of the American Association of Suicidology, president of the Association of Psychologists in Academic Health Centers, and president-elect of the Society for Clinical Child and Adolescent Psychology. In addition to her active involvement in professional training and research mentorship activities, she is active in public policy initiatives related to youth suicide prevention.

Laurel K. Leslie, MD, MPH, is the associate director of the Center on Child and Family Outcomes at Tufts–New England Medical Center. Dr. Leslie's research interests focus on the identification and treatment of developmental and mental health needs of children and adolescents across the health, mental health, and school sectors; the impact of guidelines and policy initiatives on youth service use and outcomes; and collaborative models of care across sectors that incorporate the child and family as active participants in care. Dr. Leslie's expertise in behavioral and developmental pediatrics is recognized nationally; work with the American Academy of Pediatrics and National Initiative on Children's Healthcare Quality includes development of an attention-deficit/hyperactivity disorder (ADHD) tool kit; the Education in Quality Improvement for Pediatric Practice interactive, Web-based continuing medical education module on ADHD; the Pediatric Leadership Alliance; and the American Board of Pediatrics' current Residency Review and Redesign Project.

Gabriele S. McCormick is a writer, editor, and former staff member of the American Psychological Association. She has collaborated on books, reports, and journal articles dealing with women's issues, particularly depression and women's health, and issues affecting children, youth, and families. She coordinated the Summit on Women and Depression (2000), bringing together internationally renowned experts from a variety of disciplines to provide a state-of-the-art review of research findings, make recommendations for health policy and practice, and generate a research agenda. She also edited the resulting report. Ms. McCormick provided staff support for the Task Force on Psychotropic Medications for Children and Adolescents, the Task Force on Psychology's Agenda for Child and Adolescent Mental Health, and the Task Force on Adolescent Girls. She edited reports for these groups and coauthored *A New Look at Adolescent Girls: Strengths and Stresses: Research Agenda.* Ms. McCormick also contributed to the editing of the *Report of the Task Force on the Sexualization of Girls.*

William E. Pelham Jr., PhD, is a graduate of Dartmouth College and earned his PhD in clinical psychology from the State University of New York at Stony Brook in 1976. He is currently distinguished professor of psychology, pediatrics, and psychiatry at the State University of New York at Buffalo (UB) and director of the Center for Children and Families at UB. His summer treatment program for attention-deficit/hyperactivity disorder (ADHD) children has been recognized by the American Psychological Association (APA), the Substance Abuse and Mental Health Services Administration, and CHADD (Children and Adults With Attention-Deficit/Hyperactivity Disorder) as a model program and is widely recognized as the state of the art in treatment for ADHD. Dr. Pelham has authored or coauthored more than 275 professional papers dealing with ADHD and its assessment and treatment—psychosocial, pharmacological, and combined. He has held more than 40 research grants from federal agencies (National Institute of Mental Health [NIMH], National Institute on Alcohol Abuse and Alcoholism [NIAAA], National Institute on Drug Abuse [NIDA], National Institute of Neurological Disorders and Stroke, Institute of Education Services), foundations, and pharmaceutical companies. He has served as a consultant–advisor on ADHD and related topics to numerous federal agencies (NIMH, NIAAA, NIDA, Institute of Medicine, Office of Medical Applications of Research, and the Centers for Disease Control and Prevention) and organizations (American Academy of Pediatrics, American Academy of Child and Adolescent Psychiatry, APA, CHADD). He founded and directs the biennial Niagara Conference on Evidence-Based Treatments for Childhood and Adolescent Mental Health Problems.

John C. Piacentini, PhD, ABPP, is professor of psychiatry and biobehavioral sciences in the David Geffen School of Medicine and director of the Child OCD, Anxiety, and Tic Disorders Program at the Semel Institute for Neuroscience and Human Behavior at the University of California, Los Angeles. He received his PhD in clinical psychology from the University of Georgia and completed postdoctoral training and was a faculty member at Columbia University/New York State Psychiatric Institute. Dr. Piacentini has authored over 125 papers, chapters, and books and has received numerous National Institutes of Health and other grants addressing the etiology, assessment, and treatment of childhood anxiety and obsessive–compulsive disorder, tic disorders, and adolescent suicide. He is a founding fellow of the Academy of Cognitive Therapy and a member of the American Board of Clinical Child and Adolescent Psychology. He is also deputy editor for the *Journal of the American Academy of Child & Adolescent Psychiatry* and an editorial board member for several leading psychology journals.

Benedetto Vitiello, MD, is a psychiatrist with expertise in psychopharmacology and treatment research. He has been with the National Institute of Mental Health since 1989 and is currently the chief of the Child and Adolescent Treatment and Preventive Interventions Research Branch. He has been involved in clinical trials in various areas, including child, adolescent, adult, and geriatric psychiatry, and in patients with HIV infection. He has been part of many publicly funded clinical trials testing the effects of interventions in children and adolescents, such as the Multimodal Treatment of Children With Attention Deficit Hyperactivity Disorder, the Treatment for Adolescents with Depression Study, the Research Units on Pediatric Psychopharmacology network studies, the Preschoolers With ADHD Treatment Study, and the Treatment of Early Onset Schizophrenia Study. Dr. Vitiello has authored or coauthored about 200 scientific publications, of which about 150 appear in peer-reviewed journals.